Barbara Jay

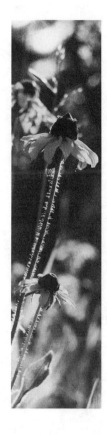

Finding Ways

Recovering From Rheumatoid Arthritis Through Alternative Medicine

Synchrony Publishing ✶ *Palo Alto, California*

Finding Ways
Recovering From Rheumatoid Arthritis Through Alternative Medicine

Copyright © 1997 by Barbara Jay Nies
ISBN 0-9653648-6-0
Library of Congress Catalog Number 96-92944

DISCLAIMER
This book is a reference work not intended to treat, diagnose or prescribe. The information contained herein is in no way to be considered as a substitute for consultation with a duly licensed healthcare professional.

Cover and interior by Troy Scott Parker, Cimarron Design
Printed in the United States of America by Gilliland Printing

Synchrony Publishing
PO Box 60205
Palo Alto, California 94306-0205

A portion of the proceeds from the sale of this book will be donated to the

AMERICAN INDIAN COLLEGE FUND

and to

CASA: CALIFORNIA COURT APPOINTED SPECIAL ADVOCATE ASSOCIATION

IN GRATEFUL HONOR OF MY TEACHER,

RALPH WALDO EMERSON,

WHO WROTE:

If the light come to our eyes, we see; else not.
If truth come to our mind,
we suddenly expand to its dimensions.

The secret of genius is to suffer no fiction
to exist for us; to realize all that we know;
in the high refinement of modern life,
in arts, in sciences, in books, in men,
to exact good faith, reality, and a purpose;
and first, last, midst and without end,
to honor every truth by use.

Contents

Acknowledgments

FOR READING AND EDITING and commenting and reassurance when my nerve failed, I thank my good and true friends: Henley Eames, Dee and Dean Morrow, Elisabeth Seaman, Adele Steinmetz, and Patricia Sussman; my beloved children, Adrienne and Kevin; and my sibling-friends, Judy, Greg, and especially Mark, who held my hand more than a sister had a right to expect.

For professional help in my recovering I thank practitioners Theresa Laehn, C.P.H.T., Sandra Kamiak, M.D., Mary Stuart, L.Ac., and Dr. Jenny Shi, O.M.D., L.Ac.

For his sensitive eye, technical skill, and his very generous and warm professionalism, I thank Troy Scott Parker of Cimarron Design.

Introduction

WHEN MEDICAL SCIENCE finally named the disease that had already distorted my life for six years, the first of many rheumatologists told me that researchers were *that* close to finding the cause of and cure for rheumatoid arthritis; that all I needed to do was to sit tight and take various prescriptions which would hold the disease at bay for the year or two—five at *most*—needed until the true and final cure was established. Above all, I was warned, in the meantime I should not fall for any of the old wives' tales I would hear, the folk remedies I might read about, the weird dietary changes that might be suggested to me, the unproven and unconventional or foreign therapies I might run across. I was told to just hang on because the cavalry was on its way.

Sixteen years later, as the cause of RA remained as elusive as ever and the treatment of last resort was failing me, and my rheumatoid arthritis with its deformity and limitation raged on, and permanent crippling threatened, and there was nothing left to lose, I dared to do the forbidden—and that has made all the difference.

Today I am over 90% symptom-free and still improving.

These pages, offered for the encouragement of people with unresponsive, progressive, debilitating rheumatoid arthritis, are excerpts from a journal of my twenty-plus-year quest for healing or cure or even long-term relief. They include some of the details of my recovering from this disease which plagues more than 2.5 million people, three-quarters of whom are women according to a 1995 publication of the Arthritis Foundation.

It is *not* my purpose to attempt to persuade RA victims whose current therapy is happily effective to change anything; this book is for the long-term victim of RA for whom no therapy has been effective and who might need to know, as I needed to know—not from a researcher but from an RA victim—that disaster does not necessarily follow stepping off the beaten medical path, especially when that path has led nowhere.

The purpose of this book *is* to offer hope to the desperate, another resort for those who have exhausted every conventional last resort. This is the book for which I searched as one after another standard medical therapy failed to relieve me of the rheumatoid arthritis which tore through my body, ravaged my joints and consumed much of my youth and vigor. May it be useful to every reader.

Accepting the Tide of Being

Faith, Standard Treatment, and Failure

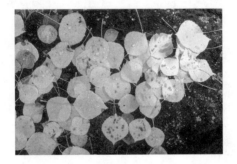

I

Accepting the Tide of Being

Wednesday, June 3, 1970

BEYOND THE LINE cut by the bulldozer as it cleared the land of scrub elms and wild strawberries to make room for our house, wild asparagus and wild grapes still flourish in undivided fields which go on for miles. Doves still mourn there in the twilight, and slugs still lurk there and conspire to ooze into my shoes when I walk among them in the morning.

The midnight sky is bright with late spring stars—in celebration of my thirty-second birthday, no doubt—as I sit on the porch step, contemplating my life and times. Birthdays, like New Year's Day and the equinoxes and solstices, are good days for stock-taking and I've been doing that all day. Bob is working late so I'm celebrating alone—except, of course, for Baby, who sleeps inside me for almost two more months, and Thor, who dozes beside me as I write by the light of two citronella candles warding off evil mosquito spirits.

Thor's pedigree is less than patrician but he compensates by being a beautiful representative of the sheltie branch of his family in his ginger-colored coat; his nervous yap betrays a less noble branch. He keeps steady company with Puff, a Great Dane who visits from the finished section of the subdivision.

Thor, and Bert and Ernie of the new children's television
program, *Sesame Street*, kept steady company with me during
the cold months I spent measuring, cutting, stitching and
installing curtains and drapes on all the windows of our nearly-
empty house. We may have a sofa with a stack of books
standing in for one leg, a forties-vintage kitchen table that lists
aport, and not one stick of furniture that was manufactured in
this half of the twentieth century, but we have nice clean walls
and splendid window coverings.

I left my day job within a month after we moved into
the house in late December to make the place livable before
Baby arrives but there's still much to do; we bought the house
partially finished and are doing the painting and staining,
grading and landscaping ourselves. I'm certainly enjoying this
change to physical labor, after so many years of sitting at a
desk—but my feet hurt.

Tuesday, June 30, 1970

> *Towels and sheets and workshirts crack and billow*
> *like sails and rumbling darkness*
> *rolls in without warning. Tornado*
> *season drops fifteen*
> *degrees in an hour and a still afternoon turns wild.*
> *My arms wrestle half-dry garments from the lines, drop*
> *clothespins like ballast as raindrops splat at*
> *twelve-inch intervals*
> *on cracked clay.*
> *I strain toward the dark house to find the wind*
> *has nailed the screen door shut and I think*
> *of lighting oil lamps*
> *in prairie cabins.*

My hips are always sore lately regardless of what I do or don't do. I hope this pain is due to pregnancy and will disappear with the arrival of Baby; I suppose it could simply be due to the fact that I'm so old to be going through my first pregnancy. I don't know what the average age at first delivery is, but I'm sure it is well below my advanced years.

I'm worried that I might have lupus like Mom since hip pain was her first symptom, and lupus does seem to run in families. She's in such pain; and her skin is so blotched and inflamed. She can't tolerate sunlight or soap or shampoo or clothing or even her own perspiration. I can't believe there's no treatment other than pain killers and steroids. I want her to look for someone who might know more than her current physician, but she won't think even of a second opinion. Maybe she could find a doctor who uses herbs or vitamins but I don't think she'll even try. And I must admit, to do that would be pretty far out of character for a woman who is in such awe of doctors that she feels she must wear a new slip for every appointment. I still don't know much about lupus but I do remember that Mrs. Leland and Edna King both died young from lupus. Sister Agnella had to stop teaching before she was fifty because of lupus. My doctor has said he'll order some tests after Baby is born.

Monday, July 6, 1970

I didn't sleep well last night and have been up since four. Thor kept me company as I picked rocks in the backyard while it was still cool. I had to set the stones carefully into my bucket so I wouldn't wake Bob. I figure if I pick one bucketful of stones each day for the next ten years, the ground might then be clear enough to sow grass seed.

I've taken some ground beef and some chickens out of the freezer to make up into casseroles to use during the first weeks after Baby comes. It's going to be hot again today so I'll close the windows and drapes on the sunny side of the house, wheel the TV into the kitchen, and Thor and I will cook and watch *Sesame Street* and *Mr. Rogers' Neighborhood.*

Tuesday, July 21, 1970

Baby Kevin Lee, who was expected to arrive around August first, came by unanticipated Caesarean section, on July seventh instead. He's healthy, noisy, and perfect!

Saturday, August 22, 1970

As if in respect for the obvious fact that the only proper activity for this sultry afternoon is sleeping, the neighborhood fauna have gone silent. On a blanket laid over the weeds under the 'thorne apple tree mercifully passed by as the bulldozer made its appointed rounds last year, Kevin naps peacefully. A sweet little breeze ruffles Thor's mane and brings him to quick attention and once again he patrols the perimeter. Thor takes his security duties more seriously now that there is a baby in the house. Inside, he stations himself under the wheeled bassinet that follows me around the house and he promises mayhem to anyone who tries to take Kevin out of his crib without going through me.

Thursday, November 12, 1970

I feel as if I'm slipping helplessly and quickly into a pit of pain and ill health. I'm really scared. My heart races. My shoulders, neck, and head are now as painful as my feet, hips, back, and hands. I have no appetite and I'm losing weight. My stomach aches whether I eat or not. I'm often dizzy and always shaky. My hair is falling out. I hyperventilate. I feel like crying all the time yet I can't cry. I haven't had a normal menstrual period since before I became pregnant. My doctors can still find no problem so have prescribed only Elavil.

Friday, December 4, 1970 — the feast of St. Barbara

Kevin crawled today! He got up on all fours on his little blanket on the floor, wiggled his bottom like a cat stalking a field mouse or a bird, advanced first a hand, then a knee, then another hand, and took off, faster and faster, chortling giddily, until he made a crash landing on his chin after traversing about two feet. All the while Thor, fascinated, studied Kevin through narrowed eyes as if he were some microscopic life form.

I saw a new internist today because I'm convinced there simply must be *something* that will actually help me and not just make me calmer and more accepting of whatever is going on in my body. But again I heard that there is no name for my combination of symptoms; that makes it unanimous among all the doctors I've consulted. Perhaps I'm paranoid on top of everything, but I have the impression that my doctors think my pains are exaggerated if not imaginary. This doctor prescribed vitamins B2 and B6.

I don't know what to do. I can't live like this. I'm barely living. I manage to take good care of Kevin but that uses up most of my energy and every day I'm worse. There's not much left for Bob, Thor, the house, or social obligations. I even hate it when people call because that takes precious energy. I'm dreading the holidays.

Tuesday, December 15, 1970

Bob's working late again so, while Kevin slept, I walked around and around and around the back yard as fluffy snowflakes floated down through perfectly still air and covered me and the trees and the house. At twenty-minute intervals I went inside to check Kevin but I just could not stay inside.

I've felt so trapped lately, by my body and my life. I feel much better when I'm outside. I would have liked to take off running and feel the wind streaming through my hair, to run for a hundred miles into blowing snow but tonight I couldn't run even a block because my feet and knees hurt so much.

I made a snowman and the cold through my mittens relieved the pain in my hands. I think I'll be sorry in the morning that I spoiled the perfection of the untouched snow but immersing myself in it has definitely lessened my discomfort tonight.

Monday, May 24, 1971

Kevin walked without support this morning and was he surprised! He'd been tooling around the family room by hanging onto furniture and crawling through the gaps but today he took the big step. I was watching him holding onto the arm of the sofa, with a strange look in his eyes, when all of a sudden he dropped both arms to his sides. He sort of rocked on his feet for a few seconds then grabbed the sofa arm, let go again, lurched forward, took three heavy steps, and plopped down on his bottom, shocked and exhausted. The look in his eyes was a strange mixture of puzzlement and delight, but he hasn't tried yet to replicate his marvelous feat.

Thursday, June 3, 1971

History repeated itself as I spent the evening of my birthday on the porch, taking stock of my life, in the company of Thor, a mourning dove I could only hear, and some mosquitoes

I could only feel as they had celebratory drinks on me. I'm thirty-three years old today. I feel twice that. I don't know what to do. Is it possible that this is all in my head? Now my gynecologist wants me to start estrogen replacement therapy because he believes I'm already in menopause. He said that hormones might help relieve the pain and fatigue and depression but he quickly adds, "No promises."

How is this possible? How can I really be menopausal at this age? I want another child.

Surveyors spent the morning staking out the lot next door and now we're facing the prospect of losing the solitude and minor wilderness that attracted us in the first place—although we knew it was inevitable. Two years ago, we chose this subdivision because it was at the northern and western outposts of suburbia but already as I drive around the area I see the first spoor of more development—orange stakes out in the middle of the fields of nowhere. How long will it be until all the open space between the little towns and bigger cities are completely colored in with one bedroom community after another?

Sunday, February 27, 1972

The twenty-foot juniper in the back yard, the largest of the two trees spared by the bulldozer when this land was cleared, is always majestic but tonight, sheathed in ice, its beauty takes my breath away. All day I watched snow light on her wide branches then disappear as if absorbed by her blackish needles; then when the air temperature dropped this evening and the snow was succeeded by heavy mist, I watched the thin shell of ice envelope her. Now, after midnight, the juniper glows silver, as if from inside, as if from her soul, in the vague moonlight.

I haven't seen a doctor yet but I know I'm pregnant; I remember the signs. I've stopped taking the Premarin because I doubt that a fetus would benefit from extra estrogen. How is it possible that a menopausal woman can so easily become pregnant?

Wednesday, March 15, 1972

It's official—I'm pregnant. Baby Too is due around the twenty-third of September.

Monday, May 1, 1972

Kevin and I planted salvia and dusty miller and leaf lettuce in front of the porch this morning but my visit to the obstetrician this afternoon sucked all joy from that and everything else we did today.

I tried to arrange for a tubal ligation after Baby Too comes but it appears that this is not a choice I may make on my own. It seems that I must first secure my husband's written permission, with his signature witnessed by two people. Then I must submit this document to my physician, who will submit it to the hospital where the tubal ligation would take place.

A board at the hospital will then apply a formula to the facts of my case—my age, the number and ages of my living children, the number and dates of stillborn children or miscarried pregnancies, my general state of health, my obstetrician's recommendation and, of course, my husband's permission, and, oh yes, my reasons for wanting a tubal ligation—to decide whether they will permit the procedure to be done immediately after the birth of Baby Too. It seems my body and its functions are not mine to control. It seems that control is anyone's *but* mine.

I feel like a cow who can be required to calve and lactate without even an inquiry into my thought on the matter. Thank goodness Bob is in complete sympathy with my reaction to this revolting situation.

Friday, June 2, 1972

The powers have spoken; I may have a tubal ligation.

Saturday, June 3, 1972

Not even the sun is up yet but I can't sleep. It's wonderfully cool and pleasant here on the porch with my coffee. Some ambitious night birds are chattering busily away, laying out their plans for the day, I suppose. Writing in this gray light is barely possible but mysterious and even somehow a little naughty. What have I come to that I am thrilled by so little?

I'm thirty-four today. I miss writing these notes to myself but I'm so busy these days that I rarely have time for more personal indulgence than the minimum standard hygiene. I may never find time to write once Baby Too arrives but, right now, the world looks good. The sun's on his way, the rest of the household sleeps, and I've already had a shower.

The pain, once predictable and constant, now hits and runs. My feet might be unbearably painful for awhile, then they will feel better as my hips, or my shoulders, or my knees, start hurting. Sometimes the pain is excruciating; at other times it's only annoying. Sometimes it's constant; yet often it's fleeting.

Saturday, September 2, 1972

Adrienne Joanna was born yesterday afternoon. She's normal, healthy, and beautiful. My tubes have been tied but my reproductive system, awash in post-partum hormones, is in full function, generating cramps and twinges, secretions, sensations and urges I haven't felt before. The Caesarean incision, closed with conventional sutures as well as metal staples that look like the devices used to secure Ace bandages, stings and burns now that all local and general anesthetic has worn off. And now all the other pain I'd almost forgotten about is back in force.

Wednesday, September 6, 1972

We're home. I'm *glad* I have a prescription for Librium because, right now, the only reason I can think of to live is to raise these two children. The pain has now spread to my pelvis. I am utterly depressed. Fortunately, I know that post-partum depression ends—I've passed this way before. But the physical pain seems unending.

Tuesday, November 7, 1972

I finally have a diagnosis for one of my symptoms. It seems that the pelvic pain and the back pain result from a condition called *condensens ilia* (pelvic deposits) which occasionally follows pregnancy in some women. There is no treatment except pain-killers. The orthopedist who ordered the x-rays gave me a prescription for butazolidin-alka and offered me a prescription for yet another tranquilizer to help me deal with my responsibilities and with the pain; he seemed surprised when I declined.

New Year's Eve

Another ice storm has made the roads treacherous so I'm glad we're not out tonight. The trees in the fields are bowed under the weight of the glaze of ice and the juniper has bowed her head toward the east.

Everything is still now. The children sleep upstairs, Bob and Thor breathe lightly in their sleep on the other side of the room, and the log in the fireplace is sighing its last. I'm very tired but I want to savor this stillness, this poise, as long as I can, and store it up for the days ahead. It's been an uphill year. I think I'll sit here until midnight to welcome the new year.

Wednesday, January 31, 1973

The first snow in six days spreads another coat over the broad expanse of brilliant white lighting up the night beyond the back windows. Only the pulsing glow of a hot-burning log in the fireplace moves and the only sound I hear is Thor's breathing next to me. It's not even ten yet and I've already been writing for more than an hour. The children have both been asleep since shortly after seven.

It's been an unbelievable day! Adrienne fussed for about an hour at lunch time, then fell asleep and slept for three hours, the first daytime nap she's taken in four months. I almost didn't know what to do with myself when both children were sleeping at the same time in the middle of the day. There are many things I might have done but I spent the time reading more of *Let's Have Healthy Children* by Adele Davis. I want to understand a lot more than I do about nutrition.

After Adrienne awoke, peaceful and alert, she poked and giggled at the mobile hanging over the rolling crib as I talked to her about the beef stew I was preparing for dinner. She looked as if she was taking mental notes as I explained the relative merits of larger and smaller pieces of onion and of the thickening power of potato starch. When I turned her over on her tummy she bobbed her little head up and down, like a turtle, trying to see over the top of the bumper pad. She spent hours this afternoon looking around, as if she had just arrived from Planet X and found us all very odd indeed.

Thursday, May 17, 1973

The lot next door was shaved bald by a yellow bulldozer as soon as the frost ban was lifted more than a month ago, and heavy equipment was once again permitted on subdivision roads. Tonight a power shovel waits still for an operator even though all morning hard-hatted men trudged through the sea of mud the lot had become, and shaded their eyes, and pointed and gestured to each other. I notice that four other lots on our street were staked out sometime last week so by fall we'll have neighbors.

Sunday, July 15, 1973

Bob's folks and their friends, Harvey and Elizabeth, were here for the afternoon. Harvey dowsed a water well for us so Bob will start that project soon. He's also planning to dig some fifteen-foot silver maples to move into the back yard during the winter.

Monday, August 20, 1973

We returned yesterday from a whirlwind trip to visit my brother in Houghton and Bob's relatives in northern Wisconsin.

Northern Michigan is so beautiful with its forests and lakes and rivers and waterfalls and wide open spaces between small old towns which date back to the copper-mining era. We visited Lake Manganese and the Keewenaw Peninsula which juts out into icy Lake Superior and had lunch at a restaurant which had been in its glory days the Calumet Opera House. Street after street of identical company housing and miles-long mounds of tailings are constant reminders of the days when the mines flourished. Now the copper is all gone and the mines are filled with water and the main industries are tourism and, some locals joke, alcoholism.

In the farmland of northern Wisconsin I was immediately at home. I think I'd love to live on a farm. Aunt Faye bakes bread and pastries, as pretty as any I've ever seen in a commercial bakery, in a wood-burning cast iron stove. She has crocks of pickles in brine, at various stages of cure, lined up along a wall in her warm kitchen. Her pantry is full of jarred peaches and plums and tomatoes, green beans and peas and beets, jams, jellies, honey, pickled watermelon rind and pickled cauliflower, corn relish and pickle relish and grape conserve. She sends home-made candy to the relatives at Christmas.

Aunt Faye's laundry flutters from a long line stretched almost to the barn where a milking herd meditates in the evening after a hard day at pasture. She shades her eyes with her hand as she watches a haying crew sweat a morning's work into the barn, then serves a mid-day meal of meatloaf, corn she picked this morning, potato salad, green beans, coleslaw, homemade bread, and gingerbread with hand-whipped cream.

The roads of northern Wisconsin smell like vinegar. The odor comes from a liquid waste product from nearby pulp mills which is spread on the gravel county roads to keep the dust down. The afternoons are hot. The fields are carpeted with golden stubble and manned by armies of drying corn shocks. The nights are surprisingly cold. The uncles speculate about when the first frost will appear and talk about the years in which they'd already had snow by this day in August.

There's a dark side to farming, I know. I've read *Grapes of Wrath* and articles about the vanishing American farmer. But I prefer to think of the romance of living close to an always-benevolent earth and to write haiku about my tourist impressions.

> *Husky green jacket*
> *Hides rows of yellow teeth*
> *Making fresh popcorn.*

Saturday, September 1, 1973

Rainy is a year old today and she took her first long series of steps. She smiles and giggles all the time and, when I took the kids for the $2.98 photograph special at Sears, she charmed the socks off the photographer with her girlish poses and impish smiles! It's hard to believe that she is the same little girl who cried with colic for nine or ten hours a day for four long months.

Friday, September 21, 1973

I'm dead tired. It's past midnight, thus actually Saturday, but I had to record for my future perusal a moment in our family life that occurred less than an hour ago:

It's an sweltering night and I'm folding diapers at the counter in the kitchen and listening to the 11 o'clock news on the television in the next room. I can barely hear the TV over the clanging and banging as Bob and his brother-in-law drive casing for an irrigation well down through the resistant clay at the back edge of the lot where Harvey had located water with his dowsing rod. They're working by the light of car headlights and I'm watching them through the open kitchen window. Thor is supervising. The children are somehow sleeping through the din.

I'm sweating; they must be sweating like race horses. We're out here in the middle of nowhere, soon to be somewhere with all the construction going on in the neighborhood. As midnight approaches, I'm still working and they're still working. We must be up at five to pick up mushrooms to freeze and a load of spent mushroom soil to use to improve the soil in our front yard before we lay sod, and we're still working. We've been working since six and we're still working. Never in my wildest unmarried dreams did I imagine I would ever work so hard!

Tuesday, January 1, 1974

Bob and the kids are still deep in sleep. Even Thor didn't stir when I stepped over him to come downstairs. There's no quiet so profound as New Year's morning quiet, I think. In a few hours, some people will start mopping up the traces of last night's celebration, or preparing to take year-end retail inventories. Others will be making plans to load up on holiday merchandise at post-holiday clearance sales, or starting up the machinery of football bowl game parties. But, for a few hours longer, silence will prevail and it's almost possible to hear the earth rotating on her axis toward sunrise.

Sunday, May 5, 1974

My fingers were cold but I spent a pleasant morning planting perennial seedlings in the raised beds we've been working on for the past weekends. I can just see the glorious masses of poppies, lupines, pinks, mums, nasturtiums, carnations...

Saturday, June 15, 1974

Kevin has been working in retail for two days now. He caught some worms in the field and had me letter this sign for him: "Worms For Sale Or Rent—You must pay me a deposit in case you forget where you left the worm." His biggest volume was in rentals because his customers couldn't see any fish in the creek so were reluctant to buy outright. His greatest profit, however, was derived from deposits which his unhappy customers had to forfeit when rented stock was returned dry or immobile. So far he's seven cents in the black but his inventory is shrinking and he can't find more worms.

Wednesday, July 3, 1974

Some of the folks from Wisconsin are visiting so I spent the evening preparing for the gathering of Bob's clan here tomorrow. We'll have barbecued beef ribs, two kinds of potato salad, sweet corn, green beans with bacon, Waldorf salad, six-bean salad, corn bread, and strawberry shortcake.

Thursday, July 4, 1974

A fun day! Everyone helped with serving and we used paper dishes so my hostess chores were minimal and I got to play badminton with Bob's young cousins whom I beat handily four games out of six! It's great to have a strong healthy body again!

Wednesday, June 4, 1975

Today Bob's folks took the kids and me to Belle Isle for a
picnic and to see the new petting zoo. I hadn't been there in
years and old memories came flooding back as soon as we
turned onto the bridge. The aquarium and flower houses all
look about the same, or a little tired maybe. The stables are
still there but I didn't see any horses. The bike rental is much
bigger than it used to be. Just like old times, the pavilion was
filled with old men playing checkers or kibitzing on the sunny
benches.

I didn't bring a notebook because it didn't occur to me
that I might have a moment to write. However, Grandma and
Grandpa wanted to take the kids to the aquarium alone so
I found myself wishing for more than a purse-fuzzy memo pad
with tissue shreds embedded in its glued spine. I rarely write
these days because the speed of our life is forever faster and
there's just no time. Once in awhile I have an idea for a verse
or an essay, and I do make a note on my desk calendar, but
I usually don't get around to developing anything. I haven't
read a book in months.

> *His chauffeur delivers him to morning*
> *checkers in the park with other*
> *vets of the American way, survivors*
> *of the fittest smokestack*
> *industry. The comrade*
> *asks brightly, "How you?"*
> *"Eatin' reg'lar," our hero beams.*

Monday, July 7, 1975

Kevin is five years old today. A few of the neighbor kids and
a couple of cousins were here for hot dogs and cupcakes at

lunch, and Grandma and Grandpa and an assortment of aunts and uncles came for dinner.

I got such a kick out of Kelly at lunch today. She obviously hears a different drummer...

Born at the age of ten, she'll be four in September.
Mincing maple seeds she asks businesslike
to borrow a pot of water
to visit for a couple bits.

She displays matter-of-factly
a recent invention—a plant-tickler:
three green toothpicks stuck in a soft bean.

Her parents had a misunderhearing she reports
her mother baked a new recipe last Farday—
turkey balls.

She finds fossils in the slag drive.
Once she stuck glops of lather in her armpits
and apologized for not shaving
the morning of tonsil surgery.

Today she made hair on her tiny cream chest
by frizzling her old Greek Grandma's hairnet
into her swim suit.

She takes Ritalin every morning
for her mother's nerves.

For the last few days my feet have been pretty sore. I hope it's due to the heat or being on them for long days and chasing

after two little kids rather than a recurrence of what I had
before.

Sunday, August 3, 1975

Memory: Family Reunion Picnic—Circa 1951

Cousins vaccinate each other with pop bottle caps
Hires, Nesbitt's, Vernor's and
mooch desserts
angelfood with lemon frosting so acid it feels cold
chocolate cupcakes with chocolate frosting in a tan shoebox
devilsfood with maple meringue and chopped walnuts.

Fat uncles gone gray like mushrooms
play flies and grounders in the boiling sun, sprawl
spread-legged against split-log benches, curse
and redden, gulp beer
threaten one-armed push-ups.

Little boys swing careless, too high
and dive into rusty pine duff nearly
put their eyes out. Darling daughters
in missing barrettes and sailor dresses, scuff
First Communion Mary Janes, share sacred secrets.

Combatant aunts
in pastel sundresses
over girdles
under straw hats
with grosgrain bands and streamers
behind round brown sunglasses
bug-eye each other's tables.

The Best Way To Eat a Broken Apple Pie

Hunch shoulders, plant elbows
plunge fork
into vanilla ice cream
a little from the shoulder, next
a fingertip in the juice all
flecked with cinnamon and maybe
clove
offer a toast—mmmmmmm is always nice if
the lower crust is soggy
scrape the slippery lining
into the residue of the cream then
consecrate the dense beige shell in one piece
on trembling fingertips
in tribute to the culinary gods.

Monday, September 1, 1975

Rainy is three years old today. The grandmas and grandpas
and some of the aunts and uncles and cousins celebrated here
yesterday with the usual dinner and gifts. Today Rainy was
feted again by Kev, cousins Michael and Bradley, and four
neighborhood children, with hot dogs, cupcakes, lemonade,
and lots of running around and shouting and no tears at all as
eight kids "shared" the opening of the gifts.

Historical Marker

A wooden footbridge
painted this season
(OSHA yellow)
faces foreign granite
there to dedicate this minor island
to commemorate Our Fallen Warriors.

Gray gazebos, tumble-
down fireplaces, wither
among arbors failing
along a lane of native limestone
erupting through gray subsoil.

Queen Anne's lace and devil's paintbrush
line a file of concrete squares
the easternmost etched 1945 and
eight cracked panels naked in the sun
gather weary 'round a rusted flagpole
a bronze Lest We Forget.

My soul revived last week in Alpena. We spent entire
days in the clear waters of Long Lake and Lake Huron, getting
intimate with the flora and fauna. The water felt so good on
my feet which have been worse lately. Kevin loved sinking
ankle deep into the reedy muck at the water's edge and Rainy
hated it.

The kids thought sleeping in the same bed was great fun,
and having Sugar Corn Pops for breakfast and sparklers every
evening after dark. We read at least two long stories each day
and caught butterflies and searched, with some luck, for
fireflies and bats.

One day we walked out to a lighthouse on a limestone spit
and our footsteps sounded like beats on a planet-size drum. We

watched a black wall of rain blow across Lake Huron from its Canadian shore and we ran for the car when we were pelted with hailstones. I could hardly run because my feet hurt so badly.

The best part of the week was the fact that I wrote every morning and every night. With few chores and no television, time seemed limitless. I nearly filled a new green spiral notebook with verse and scribbles and I outlined a short story. I wrote in my journal. Writing is my drug of choice.

Wednesday, September 3, 1975

Kevin started kindergarten this morning and announced, when Rainy and I met him in the schoolyard at noon, that he didn't think he'd be going back because he didn't know how to read well enough.

Friday, October 31, 1975 — Halloween

A warm hazy Indian Summer day. After we walked Kevin to school, Rainy and I took a ride down Halstead Road and cut a bunch of sumac for the vase next to the fireplace. The burgundy of the sumac clusters is so vivid and the texture is the silkiest velvet. I was shocked out of my bliss by lines of those ominous orange stakes springing up like the proverbial toadstools after a rain along that dusty lane.

After school we went to the cider mill which was swarming with moms and kids on similar mission. We got a couple of gallons of cider but since they only fry donuts on the weekends we had to make do with maple sugar candy.

Just as the littlest kids were starting out on their trick-or-treat rounds this evening, an almost imperceptible mist began falling so, by the time Bob brought Kevin and Rainy back to

the house, Kevin's crepe paper leprechaun costume was
bleeding green down his neck and hands and into his shoes.
I'd made Rainy's witch costume out of waterproof nylon so
she was dry as a little bone.

If the number of caramel corn balls I passed out this
evening is any indication, this subdivision is full to overflowing.
Only a few years ago we were living at the edge of civilization
and now we're somewhere in a vast sea of people. Sad.

Tuesday, August 24, 1976

We spent a restful week camping in the cool pine and oak
forest beyond the dunes on the Canadian shore of Lake Huron.
Now, back in the heat at home we are having an irrigation
well *drilled*. Bob's efforts to *drive* a well didn't yield anything
because, as he discovered too late to avoid all that sweaty labor,
the water table here is well below a hundred feet, too deep for
a hand-driven well. The dowser was right about the location
but wrong about the depth. If we want a well it will have to
be drilled by machine.

The drill rig rises twenty feet into the air as monster bits
are lubricated with water pumped from a tank truck. The
drillers are reduced to mere muddy body weight as they
straddle the great iron tools into position. They wear the blank
mask of machine-induced deafness and oily prime climbs the
muddy denim wicks their legs have become.

Engines ease a stainless steel phallus in and out, in and
out of the reluctant earth. A birth canal is slowly opened and
a vertical spasm of mud turns into a stony column of space.

Shallow black earth smells like birth
false labor at twenty feet—
sand
and
brown clay
blue clay
gray clay
stillborn
hardpan

the din
the vibration
the twisting
the ramming
the ringing
the banging
the clanging
drive deeper
and deeper
pound faster
and faster
strike harder
and harder

then water
cold water
stands grandly
and sacred
in glory
above us.

While we were up north I reaffirmed my desire to write—
but doesn't everyone want to write? I know how to write, sort
of, but I don't know how to go about *becoming a writer,* and I

certainly don't know whether I can write anything publishable. Does that matter? Still I've had this hit-and-run dream for such a long time that it seems I should earnestly attempt to fulfill it or exorcise it from the closet of spirits that haunt me.

Thursday, September 2, 1976

Whereas Kevin is only in first grade, Adrienne started college today, according to her. I registered her in the child care program at the Oakland Community College so I could enroll in a creative writing class. It's been so long since I've had time to read and I find now that I'm hungry to get back to it and ready to start writing regularly.

I woke up again this morning with a stinging pain at the base of my neck. I suppose it's from sleeping on a different bed, then returning to my own bed. My feet are still hurting. If I'm not better in a week I'll see a doctor. I'm assuming that what's happening now is unrelated to the other siege that ended more than two years ago.

Sunday, October 5, 1980

In October of 1976 an internist tentatively diagnosed my problem as rheumatoid arthritis and passed me on to a rheumatologist who confirmed the diagnosis and sent me home with a packet of materials from the Arthritis Foundation.

I read that rheumatoid arthritis is a form of arthritis which causes inflammation of the lining of the joints or internal organs or both. The inflammation causes pain and stiffness, and can also cause debility and deformity. I read that three-quarters of the people who have RA are women and about one percent of the population of the US has RA which usually begins in the early adult years. The cause is not known although there is current research to establish whether it results from a viral or bacterial infection, or is a manifestation of a genetic or immune system defect. The Arthritis Foundation warns against losing valuable treatment time to quackery and outlines the accepted treatments and medications. There is no cure.

I learned that the first line of treatment is saturation doses of an anti-inflammatory agent—aspirin in my case. I was instructed to begin with two aspirin tablets every four hours around the clock. Each day I was to increase each dose by one tablet until I experienced ringing in my ears and then to drop back by one tablet at each dose until the ringing stopped. By this method I took thirty-six aspirin on day five when the ringing started. I dropped back to thirty tablets on day six, but the ringing continued and I became nauseated. On day seven, my saturation dosage of twenty-four aspirin tablets, which I have taken daily since then, was established.

The aspirin therapy did reduce the pain but it did nothing to stop or even slow the disease. An odd spread developed between toes three and four on both feet and my AA-width shoes had to be replaced with C-width shoes. My hands stayed hot, red, and swollen. I developed a duodenal ulcer from the aspirin and got to the point of surreptitiously swigging liquid antacid directly from the bottle that I always carried in my handbag—my version of bag wine.

If RA made the first of many random visits in 1970, and finally revealed itself to laboratory science in 1976, it moved in and took over with a vengeance in the summer of 1979, a summer of tears, on the occasion of my first-ever, first post-divorce separation from my children as they left for a week's vacation with their dad.

Sleep was impossible. My shoulders would clutch and my ribs would clamp and jolt me awake as soon as I dropped off to sleep. My hips and knees throbbed night and day. I was too weak to make a sandwich *and* wash the plate. The taut skin of my swollen hands and feet itched and stung. The only shoes I could bear to wear were sponge rubber thongs. The pressure of ordinary clothing was too much. My eyes burned, my heart raced. I hallucinated from lack of sleep.

I continued taking aspirin and started working in private and group psychotherapy to eliminate any unconscious psychological need for this disease. I could barely drive to the therapy sessions because holding the wheel tortured my hands and shoulders. I became terrified of driving itself. I had nightmares of falling over the edges of cliffs, of falling off bridges, of being hunted down in the dark by someone I didn't know.

The children returned from their week with their dad and I could barely care for them. On the contrary, that first summer they were virtual hands and feet to me as descending the basement stairs and doing certain chores such as changing bed linen became impossible. At ages eight and six, they were willing enough and learned to do more and more of the household chores.

If I was depressed earlier, I was nearly suicidal as, one by one, common activities became so painful I avoided all but the most vital. I wept in pain and in self-pity and hated myself for both. Fortunately, since we had only moved into our freshly-painted, spotless and much smaller house in March, the minor housekeeping of which I was capable did not really show and I began improving before the children returned to school that September.

By fall, our life was returning to normal and gradually a healthier, more appropriate division of labor was restored. We did all the things that most other families did—Cub Scouts, Brownies, field trips, family visits, picnicking. We adopted two four-month-old Lab-Cocker litter-mates from the county animal shelter and they became our babies and the biggest nuisance and most terrible responsibility and greatest joy in our lives!

I worked as a bookkeeper and occasionally wrote a bit of verse or an essay. I dated a little but there was not enough energy for family life and a romantic life as well. I tried to swim at the local Family Y one evening when the children were with their dad, and was shocked to discover that not only could I no longer hoist myself out of the water using only my arms and shoulders, I couldn't even comfortably use the metal ladder. And the cold water made my joints even more painful and stiff.

I continued seeing the rheumatologist and taking aspirin. I continued taking antacids. I continued in group therapy and, despite the pronouncements of the Arthritis Foundation, I continued to expect to recover soon from this inconvenient disease. After all, I had a glorious childhood to provide for my children and, of course, I hoped to become the Great American Novelist.

Sunday, November 2, 1980

> *All that's left are poised patterns, stencils*
> *of the sweet colors of summer and scent.*
> *Autumn's vibrancy now lies drab in rags, light*
> *and shine hibernates in leaden sight, united*
> *by generic days, generic nights.*

This morning is stilled by frost. It reminds me. Of voids, rejections, of constant silent and spoken messages to be still, soundless, undemanding. Any morning is a blank sheet of paper and the very sunrise creates tension as it invites, teases, requires, demands—reminds.

The soul can rest in sleep while its processes lie unfueled by daylight. It can integrate, heal, assimilate, metabolize. It can open its eyes and trust itself in dream. But by day the soul is a sponge, wringing out memories, sopping up hope.

The aspirin alone did nothing to control the aggression of RA so I've been having gold salts injections since April. By now I should be on the maintenance regime of an injection every three or four weeks. But each time I try to increase the interval beyond two weeks I soon worsen so, obviously, these gold salts injections have been helping somewhat. Nonetheless the damage continues.

I can almost hold the pain at bay with the aspirin but the side-effects are very much a problem. My hearing has deteriorated from so much aspirin and I pop antacid tablets for my ulcers like some people pop candy.

Now my fingers are starting to deviate to the outside of my hands and when I sleep they clench like claws. I use resting splints at night to prevent the clawing and to ease the pain in my wrists. I had a paraffin bath at the doctor's office once, and it was very soothing, but to duplicate that at home would be too elaborate, too time-consuming, and too dangerous for such temporary relief. I do range-of-motion exercises morning and evening but I'm still losing ground.

I did much better during the few months when Dr. Carter was giving me prophylactic penicillin injections in addition to the Myochrysine. Unfortunately, she moved to Florida after she had been treating me for only three months and my current rheumatologist believes that such use of penicillin can't possibly be effective so he won't even try it. (It seems there have been no double-blind studies to pronounce real and genuine my experience of this therapy. Maybe I imagined it...)

This new doctor says that any effect I felt was only that of a placebo. I don't care if it was! I'll take anything, placebo or snake oil or eye of newt, that will safely work! Let him be a purist with his *own* diseases—I want anything that will help whether it's scientific or not! I'm getting sick of doctors acting like my body and my pain is just the inanimate field on which they're amusing themselves, or aggrandizing themselves, with an inconsequential game.

Fortunately, I'm showing no side-effects from the gold salts itself and I do have the promise of corrective surgery and artificial finger and toe joints if the damage continues. And I *can* earn a living and meet most of my family and social obligations even though I'm always in pain and always exhausted. I regret not maintaining my journal more regularly but I just haven't had the energy and most of the time I've been too depressed to care.

Saturday, July 4, 1981 — Independence Day

> *At a rock concert I buy*
> *a plastic flag from a paunchy vet with brown*
> *edged teeth. I don't believe*
> *in nationalism or*
> *war or begging or*
> *theft I believe in*
> *rock and the spirit of carnival.*

I can't believe that my health has been stable for more than six months now. Things are looking up!

Although I've gotten out of the habit of writing in my journal I've been doing enough other writing to compensate. Two of my short stories and five short poems were accepted by *The Arts Objectively,* a magazine devoted to the ideas of Ayn Rand and her philosophy of Objectivism. Maybe I'll write the Great American Novel yet! Hope springs eternal...

Halloween 1981

Kev, Mr. Battlestar Galactica himself, and Rain, the blue fairy princess, went out trick-or-treating with our neighbors, but they got cold after a few blocks and came home to inspect and sample their collections. More than a hundred trick-or-treaters came to the door this evening!

As always, I regret not making more frequent journal entries but these days I'm too wrapped up in other writing, submitting, reading rejection notices, etc. I should force myself to write in my journal at least once a week. But "Thou shalt not should on thyself," says Lee Shulman, my therapist.

I've been feeling trapped with neighbors so close and no ungroomed natural life nearby so, after due deliberation, I put the house up for sale after school resumed, and this week I took four vacation days and found a semi-rural place where the kids and the dogs and I will have some open space.

Sunday, January 3, 1982

I am definitely in the midst of a remission! Definitely!

Sunday, February 10, 1982 — in Wixom at last!

We've been here over a week but I don't quite feel here yet. Maybe it's because the former occupants didn't move out until the day before we moved in. I think a house needs some time to be unoccupied, some white space between occupations, for old energies to dissipate, to float away, to escape by osmosis through exterior walls.

Daily snowfall has made it difficult to keep the driveway clear enough to get in and out each day. I've taken the last of my vacation time to get settled here; I've gotten a lot done but we're certainly not settled. The biggest chore has been dispatching the ghosts of cigar smoke past that cling to every surface.

I've been feeling better and better. I'm still having gold salts injections every other Wednesday and I'm still taking twenty-four aspirin daily, so I still have my ulcer, but I think I'm going to suggest to my doctor that it might be time to try again to wean myself from both medications even though there are still diminishing problems

Sunday, March 7, 1982

Once a winter in Michigan
the world turns to glass and
children, poets, make trails and angels
and search for red penguins and snowbuds and rainbows
    in the yard
and the ordinary diamond star
behind the white moon stuck at ten o'clock
who sprinkled silver semen
and sired the storm.

One secret night
in every blackberry winter
diamond glazes all and morning,
induced by the drowning sun,
delivers spring.

Sunday, May 2, 1982

We have added another member to our family, a black kitten
named—what else?—Licorice. Rain got her from her new
friend across the road and she's just been weaned (the kitten,
not the friend). This morning Licorice managed to find her
way from Rain's bed, down the hall and into my room, up a
stack of books, onto a basket of unfolded laundry, onto a chair,
and from thence onto my bed. I didn't awaken and tend to
her needs soon enough so she summoned me by squatting on
my forehead and biting the little divider thing at the bottom
of my nose (septum?) with her needle-like teeth. I moved right
smartly after that. The dogs watch her like they watch ants and
Blackie loves to wash her with her tongue as if she's a newborn
puppy. On the other hand, Licorice is still circumspect
about Fuzzy and Blackie and she lets them know when their
advances are unwelcome by hooking their juicy black noses
with sharp claws.

Sunday, June 6, 1982

It's still a little cool by my standard but the kids seem perfectly
comfortable playing sock ball (with a sock full of beach sand)
in Proud Lake, while I drink coffee at a picnic table and watch
Japanese beetles mate (I think that's what they're doing).
Twelve teeny legs twitch some for two or three seconds but,
otherwise, neither moves for a goodly time…eventually he
appears to be slipping a little, perched as he is on her tiny
brown shell, and he hitches himself up some…Instantly! they
begin rolling wildly, like a spastic nutmeat, tick-ticking across
the table, gyrating with frantic abandon, popcorning over the
Sunday funnies, a rollicking, frolicking dicot joyous in the
dance of life, doubling and redoubling supercharged springing
energy, pirouetting dizzily on end and spinning together like a
firecracker!!!…Suddenly! with exquisite aim, he shoots out a

thread-like leg and clamps powerfully onto the edge of the folded newspaper…they hang, coupled, in mid-air…she swoons as he clamps his other five legs more tightly around her and, lo, what fine tremors shudder his wanton little body! They drop to the table as all his legs go flaccid. He lands on his back, shrivelled, atrophied, dried out, spent…she stretches and brushes the air from her eyes…

We finished painting the basement walls yesterday. I never thought I'd be able to do anything so strenuous again. No, that's not quite true. I did believe I'd recover from this disease; it was my *doctors* who said I'd probably never be able to do such things again.

Labor Day 1982

The last holiday of the summer and an especially welcome one to me because, since I used up my vacation time early in the year in making the move, I've only had holidays away from work since February.

I played badminton this morning for the first time in years; I'm not as good at it as I once was—yet. I also mowed part of the side yard with a hand mower. I'll never again take such ordinary abilities for granted.

Thinking about Labor Day, as I went about my household chores with that special leisure that a long weekend offers (or so it says in the ladies' magazines), brought to mind the fiction and fact surrounding my post-divorce return to the paid labor force. Let the truth be told: I loved being a full-time homemaker but I lost wage-earning capacity—*and* the potential for long leisurely weekends—during those years when I was "home with the kids" and returning to the salaried work force has not been fun, fulfilling, or lucrative.

Sunday, January 2, 1983

> *We've been through death*
> *of parents, death*
> *of a marriage or two*
> *somehow we don't seem to flame like we used to do*
> *now that we know*
> *how little we know*
> *we've lived*
> *up to some of the dreams*
> *some of the nightmares too.*

A heavy mist hangs over the early morning. As if underwater, the tracery of leafless trees looks like ice coral. A faint freeway sound, muffled by frost, could be the sound of distant submarine engines propelling this white planet softly through a vast water. It's still, absolutely still—no birds, no lights, no precipitation. Breaking the drama, a lush Irish Setter, makes his rounds of mailbox posts in a cloud of steamy breath.

Sunday, February 6, 1983

I am despondent. I've been flaring since shortly after Christmas. I've been off gold salts injections for several months because I developed lesions in my mouth; now my doctor says I can't resume gold salts therapy so I'll try penicillamine and continue with the aspirin as usual. I feel beaten. I can't believe it has come back with such vehemence, especially after months of nearly normal health.

Now that I'm so limited again, Rain and Kev and I have devised a system of dividing up the chores which somehow gives them the happy illusion that they're doing less when they're actually doing more. Whereas under our old system I would assign a task or two to each child each day, under the new system each child is the "slave," who must do chores and "gofer" duty, only on alternating days. The non-slave child not only has no household responsibilities at all, except in the case of a genuine emergency, but also has the prerogative of choosing TV programs, treats, etc.. Somehow, the days off make the work seem less and the choices more privileged. This makes me feel a *little* better about the fact that Kev and Rain are required to do much more than most children.

Sunday, March 6, 1983

Drizzle dampened most of yesterday as I went to the bank and the supermarket, and later made my way through the laundry but, since all week long the weather forecast promised a warming trend and speculated about the possibility of an early spring, the hope in my heart stayed dry. However, the temperature began to drop at sundown and the drizzle continued. At about eight I closed the drapes over the black windows and we settled into television and popcorn and disappointment.

At about eleven, after Kev and Rain had gone to their rooms, as I turned off the television I heard a tinkling sound outside. I parted the drapes to investigate and saw another universe! A fantasy landscape created by frozen drizzle that was somehow both falling and suspended in the night air.

The trees and the shrubs were all splayed into gigantic glassy flowers as the heavy ice pressed each branch individually earthward. There was no wind yet, with the television silent, the atmosphere was filled with the crackling sound of ice breaking apart, clinking, shattering, bouncing off the slick surface of the crusted snow, the sounds of the expansion and contraction of all the solid matter in that world.

The continuing ice sounds, and the memory of the glass vision outside, made it difficult for me to fall asleep but when I awoke this morning, I wondered if I only imagined the storm, because all traces of ice were gone, the sun was beaming, and snow melt puddled the driveway.

Friday, April 8, 1983

The penicillamine is helping my joints but my mood has been black and my energy low. On days when the children are with their father, I've been going to bed as soon as I've had something to eat and have talked on the phone with them.

Today spring seems to have arrived and brought renewed hope with it. I haven't felt like writing for months but today I do. My appetite for food has returned as well. I've been eating only a bowl of soup for most dinners but this evening I couldn't eat enough and it all tasted so wonderful! Everything is absolutely delicious to the truly hungry.

Usually, frozen corn on the cob, in uniform factory-determined lengths, appears so frequently on our table year-round that we no longer need crave, after a long and cornless winter, silky warm ears fresh from an August stalk. We rub so many elbows, of the animal and vegetable and mineral varieties, in so many ways that we rarely have occasion to anticipate the exquisite pleasures of simple human contact, of periodic abundance after seasons of deprivation.

Like everyone I know, I have levelled many of the peaks and back-filled many of the valleys in my life. Still I haven't derived much real pleasure from my year-round seventy-two-degree environment. I love change more. I appreciate frigid months and weighty clothing after the steam and liberty of a tropical season. I feel the lightening of spring the first day I decline to wear snow boots. I want to plunge my whole heart into the doldrums of summer so I can fully feel frost when it bites. Ebb and flow, yin and yang…

Saturday, June 11, 1983

Kev and Rain learned to ride Steven's and David's Moped today at Lucy's, where we spent the day. They have chickens now and I think Kev was getting a bright idea about getting one himself so I ever-so-casually mentioned our moratorium on animal acquisition. We had a few chickens for awhile when I was a kid and I know that they are a definite challenge.

I wish Lucy had a daughter so she and Rain could grow up together as Lucy and I did. We were closer to each other than we were to our sisters and I still cherish her friendship even though these days we only get together once or twice a year.

Saturday, June 18, 1983

Our population grows. From Sunshine Rabbit Ranch, we adopted a bunny named Buttercup who lives in a long-legged hutch constructed by the master carpenter, Kevin. Buttercup shares the garage with the dogs who live in their own four-by-four-by-eight plywood cabin, also designed and constructed by the same architect. The dogs and the bunny all do well together in their respective houses, although we don't tempt fate by taking Buttercup out of her hutch when the dogs are close by. Licorice, who I'm afraid will never be a contender for Miss Congeniality, is, as usual, another story.

After Buttercup had been with us for awhile, and having no real idea whether putting her in the same room with Lickie was prudent, we decided to test the possibilities by supervising their meeting in the bathroom with the door closed.

We brought Buttercup in first and let her hop around and sniff while Rain coached her from the edge of the tub. After Buttercup settled down, Kev brought Lickie in. Lickie assessed the situation from the neutral corner where Kev had placed her and then, in one leap across the tiny room, she spread-eagled herself over Buttercup's back, and rode that terrified bunny, yee-ha rodeo-style, around and around the room until we frantic spectators could devise a plan to separate them without drawing anyone's blood.

Sunday, November 27, 1983

Snow. Winter. Another ending. Another uncle's funeral. Since Grandpa Hooper's death when I was in grade three, I have attended the funerals of fifteen members of my family. The snow dusting our house, the trees and shrubs in the yard outside is the same snow dusting all the graves of all the relatives in Sacred Heart Cemetery, Mount Olivet Cemetery, Resurrection Cemetery.

My feet feel as if I'm walking on sharpened stones and it's difficult to conceal the discomfort and walk normally. It's very clear now that I'll need to have surgery to remove the excess tissue and mineral deposits of which these stones are made.

Sunday, February 5, 1984

In this area of feral fields and retired barns, "Free Kittens" signs and velvety-black Burmese-type cats like Lickie abound, so we weren't at all surprised to find a tiny version, complete with fleas and countable ribs, on our front porch when we arrived home one Sunday evening late last July. She was so tiny and young we couldn't figure out how she had climbed the steps to the porch or, since she was obviously not old enough to be weaned, how she had survived long enough to lose enough weight for her ribs to show.

Rain christened her "Hyper Q.T. Bbugg" as she squatted in her saucer of milk and accidentally lapped up a little. She could spend the warm night, it was agreed, in a box on the porch—we didn't want the house or our other cats or our dogs infested with fleas—and in the morning we'd find her family. We definitely could not keep her because we already had two cats, two dogs, a bunny, and a nice little group of goldfish as well as a history of other cats, dogs, snakes, lizards, and more fish. There simply was no space, time, energy, or cash for another animal. I declared a moratorium on animal acquisition more than a year ago after we adopted Good Sam, a sweet docile white male cat whose family abandoned him in the dead of winter when they moved to Tennessee.

By Labor Day we still hadn't located Bbugg's family and she had settled in with her fleas on the porch. When she could spare the time from eating—milk, cat food, dragonflies, or whatever she could catch—she would do some milling around among whosever feet were nearby. Inevitably, as we were unloading the car, in the dark, of Labor Day picnic remnants, she got stepped on.

We actually heard the sound of tiny bones giving way and, by the time we got the porch light on, she was paralyzed but breathing. She defecated, a sure sign of imminent death, we'd heard, so we brought her inside, fleas and all, to die in peace during the night. It wasn't in any of us to hasten that process.

But she didn't die. Although we were certain it was a lost cause, we took her to the vet anyway the next morning. Fractured skull. Severe nerve trauma. She could live— probably would, with steroids for a few days and nursing for who- knows-how-long; that was the choice.

She has progressed. During those first weeks she didn't move at all so I turned her and cleaned her and fed her baby formula with a stomach tube. Then slowly, bit by tiniest bit, she learned to move her forelegs, to open her eyes, move her hind legs. She learned to travel in a tight circle by clawing the towels that were her bed sheets. She twitched the tip of her tail. One day it was obvious that she could see and hear again.

In her Christmas stocking, Bbugg received a jar of baby meat to mix with her "grunch"—soaked and mashed cat food which we fed to her with a tiny baby spoon. Her milk bottle by then was a tiny hypodermic syringe, sans needle, of course.

Now she's trying to relearn to lap milk from a saucer even though her neck isn't quite self-supporting yet. Some days her hips work and she can almost achieve a stiff-legged colt-like stance. She has a yelp for a voice and she used it for one glorious moment last week.

Home now is a microwave oven box, inside the house, sans fleas which I personally dispatched, one by one. She keeps cat's hours now, sleeping during the day and flopping around in her box at night. She tries to groom herself—and whomever is holding her. She's still making progress but she may never be normal or even able to sustain her own life. I'm not sure we made the right choice; I'm not sure we didn't. Some days she forgets to eat, and catflesh is so cheap…

My feet are getting to be more and more a problem, and the swelling, stiffness, and pain in my hands, hips, and knees fades unpredictably in and out. I have only energy enough for necessities most days. I miss writing and each day I vow to write at least a sentence or two about the day but, when bedtime comes, I have barely enough energy to brush my teeth.

I've switched doctors in order to have access to a better hospital when the time comes to have joint replacement surgery. My new doctor is willing to have me try gold salts therapy again, since the penicillamine seems not to be working any more, but he wants me to first try a drug that has just been put on the market and looks very promising.

Monday, March 5, 1984

The snow is deep, the atmosphere hangs stiff and still as a carcass in a meat locker. The days warm a little, then more snow falls to clean and reintegrate the neighborhood again. But after another stolid gray day, the edges of the snow mold into an airy crust that withers like cake icing gone to sugar.

It's getting really difficult to do justice to any part of my life. My job requires too much time and the best of my energy. The children are so active and so helpful and so demanding and so undemanding and such a joy and I'm not able to savor their evolution the way I want and the way they deserve merely by virtue of their being children. I try to hoard the very best for them. The house gets almost nothing.

My depression deepens when I think about our house. A family of any size, I'm convinced, needs someone to keep vigil at its cave, to guard its fire and husband its belongings, to keep track of its comings and goings. I can live without a constant companion but I want to be home from these wars with RA and excessive wage-earning time away from the center of my life, my house, my children.

I'm off the Oraflex after only three weeks because several deaths in Ireland have been attributed to its use. I've had lab work and everything seems okay so it doesn't appear to have hurt me. I'll be going back on Solganol and aspirin after giving my body a few weeks to rest.

My new doctor is urging me to have surgery as soon as possible to remove the damaged tissue and spurs on my insteps and to repair the damage to my toes. He also recommends immediate joint replacement on all my fingers.

Although I have scheduled appointments with a foot surgeon and a hand surgeon, I'm reluctant now to have surgery because I've been hearing lately about treating RA with diet and acupuncture. Unfortunately, I haven't been able to find a nutritionist who advocates anything other than the usual and I can't find an acupuncturist at all. Apparently they can't be licensed here so I'd have to go to another state, or even to another country, to get any other kind of treatment.

There are clinics in Europe that specialize in actually curing RA, I've read in the only book I could find on the topic, but travelling to Europe is certainly out of the question for me. I've also heard that there is an experimental procedure involving blood filtration, similar to kidney dialysis, which produces remission from RA for six or more months; this procedure costs in the thousands and is not covered by insurance. I wish I had more time and energy to spend at the library to learn if there are still more options.

Sunday, March 11, 1984

Since the ice storm of last blackberry winter, the drench of spring and its lusty, musty drying-out into cool summer, I've had little energy for living and less for writing, even about looking out on life, which is about what my life has been reduced to; I can *do* very little in the way of physical activity since most activity requires the use of at least one of my damaged or painful parts. But I did *notice* it all—the building heat, the steam of July and August and the shocking drop into the end of summer, then autumn, Indian Summer, leaden

November, transparent December and real winter and around
again. I just didn't write about it.

I'm utterly depressed. Knowing that it's mostly from RA
doesn't help much. I'm sure I could get a prescription for an
anti-depressant but I'd rather do anything else than challenge
my body and my mind with yet another chemical, however
promising, and whatever synergy it might create.

I think I'd feel better if I could find the consolation of a
religion but I've tried all the name-brand religions and they
don't work any better for me than my native Catholicism did.
I've even experimented with obscure devotions, such as those
described in *The Varieties of Religious Experience* by William
James. I've even thought of going back to the church because,
despite its toxic doctrine, I do miss the consolation of its
familiar physical and symbolic aspects.

I miss the calendar of the church, dividing time into
seasons of penitence and preparation, vigils, rejoicing, and
feasts of saints.

I miss the color and texture of the church—the chaste
expanses of starched white altar cloths lavishly edged in lace
and cutwork, surplice of priest and altar boy, the nun's coif
and wimple, the long linen communion rail cloths. I miss the
Infant of Prague statue dressed like a prince doll in *peau de soie*
and seed pearls. I miss green felt altar covers and the purple
statue covers of holy week, brown funeral candles, black and
flowerless memorial masses for the dead. I miss the enveloping
black of cassock and habit.

I miss the flags of office and honor—the biretta and miter,
the red of the cardinal, violet of the monsignori.

I miss my lost saints. I prayed to St. Barbara, my namesake
and the patron of earthly calamity such as earthquake and
volcano. I prayed to St. John Bosco, the modern patron of
students; to St. Maria Goretti, a modern Italian teenager

canonized for refusing to cooperate as she was raped and
murdered, now the patron of virginity. I prayed to St. Frances
Xavier Cabrini, the first American saint. I prayed—often—
to St. Jude, the patron of hopeless causes.

I chuckled (but discreetly) at certain saints' names—
St. Cunegunda, St. Hyppolita—and wondered why some
saints had surnames—St. Charles Borromeo, St. Francis
Borgia—and others did not. From a children's book I learned
about St. Zita who was a scullery maid and had only prunes
to eat (Holy Cinderella!). I miss St. Christopher who glowed
in the dark as he rode shotgun on the dashboards of the cars
of my adolescence.

I miss the gold of chalice, ciborium, paten, monstrance,
bells. I miss tabernacles and choirs and organs and baptistries
and holy water fonts and genuflecting.

I miss the numbers of the church—three persons in God,
seven cardinal sins, eight beatitudes, ten commandments, six
precepts, nine first Fridays, five first Saturdays.

I miss Catholic smells—like candle smoke, laundry starch,
beeswax, pine boughs filling the side altar niches at Christmas,
cabbage in convents, fish in every Catholic frying pan on all
the Fridays of my life until the law requiring Friday abstinence
from meat was rescinded.

I miss the lights of Catholicism—the red sanctuary lamp
never allowed to burn out, banks of votive lights at the side
altars, the four-foot paschal candle and its new fire at Easter
daybreak, symbolic of Jesus' resurrection from death. I miss
six tall beeswax candles in gold candlesticks and collars at
high mass or two shorter candles at low mass.

I miss May crowning, Holy Week, forty hours devotion,
retreats, days of recollection, novenas, May and October
devotions to Mary the mother of Jesus, the stations of the
cross, tre ore services of Good Friday, the Baltimore
Catechism, radio rosary crusade, Bishop Sheen telecasts.

I miss the triumphant, majestic declarations of blood and seasons, virginity and death, hope and victory, and penitence, in the silk and gold and colors and velvet of cope, stole, maniple, chasuble, tabernacle curtain.

I miss receiving communion. First Holy Communion Day was the first really important day of my life. Preparing for First Communion was like preparing for a wedding, a debut into Catholic society. Even though my dress, rayon pique with satin ribbons, was made by Grandma Nies and not by the local bridal shoppe, I knew I would be stunning when I wore it with my very full silk net veil with real artificial lilies-of-the-valley on the crown part. I hated my shoes because they were two-strap sandals (strictly for summer and/or toddlers) and they were not even voted on by me.

Almost as important as the dress and veil was the "set," a combination of medals, scapulars, holy pictures, rosary, and prayer book. The centerpiece was the prayer book. The covers of the very best prayer books were genuine mother-of-pearl all shimmering lavender and pink, and printed with a picture of a pretty Jesus with long blondish hair and halo dipping the Eucharist out of a glowing ciborium for a pretty blond girl, in a white dress and veil, kneeling before him. And on the inside of the front cover—oh, glorious beauty itself—was an arched recess of iridescent white mother-of-pearl centered with a tiny golden crucifix with a tiny white genuine imitation ivory plastic corpus!

The really best part of First Holy Communion was the stockings. Sheer, long, slinky, lustrous, cool, intimate, white, silk stockings. Stockings resting in silent dignity, enfolded in white tissue, within a pristine thin square box. Stockings to be reverently gathered on trembling thumbs and slithered slowly over the big toe, other toes, instep, heel, ankle, calf, knee, thigh, and anchored so precisely to the white eyelet garter belt. No one talked about the stockings but I think we all knew that, although it was the Eucharist that made us real Catholics, it was the stockings that made us, at age seven, *women*.

Maybe I miss most the music of my childhood faith— the sweet hymns, the noble Latin and organ music of the mass. I miss the majesty of bannered cornets playing Bach in Blessed Sacrament Cathedral. I miss the timeless Gregorian chant, square-noted on unmeasured staff on yellowed paper, "*dies irae, dies illa*—day of wrath, day of mourning." I miss the a capella exchanges between priest and soloist. I miss the clappers of Holy Saturday when the bells were silenced, and the bells. In fact, it's the *bells* I miss most of all—steeple bells, the bells of consecration, of transubstantiation, of Easter's first light, the bells of my lost faith.

Fortunately, Ralph Waldo Emerson often enough moves me, uplifts me, and inspires fresh hope into my gasping soul. His words lead me to seek further. I guess I'm experiencing a protracted crisis of faith, but I suspect my greater problem is still RA and what it's doing to not only my joints but to my glands, my brain, my spirit.

Friday, April 6, 1984

> *I need to hear your breath at night*
> *to see the soft heave of your chest*
> *the innocence of your taut eyelids.*
> *I need to smell you and feel*
> *the harshness of your soles*
> *the body silk between your fingers.*
> *Who are you?*

Wednesday, May 2, 1984

Her fall is broken
by a tired gray chair tamped
into a thready sand carpet.
Everything is compacted here, devoid
of life's little cushions and light
like her joints devoid
of the gelatinous pads that once made
possible
the bounce and snap of an unfinal life.
Now she gets shorter
daily while her jawbones surrender a certain
amount of lime
and spit, and her lengthening
earlobes betray her grudging years.

Friday, May 25, 1984

The arrangements for my surgeries are almost complete.
I'll have the first one, on my right foot, in early June, and the
other three at two-month to three-month intervals. I have
such mixed feelings but my rheumatologist and the surgeons
all think the surgeries will help a lot. I hope they're right. I
have years and years and miles and miles to go before I can
think of sleeping. I'm scared and I'm hopeful…

For now, the gala Memorial Day weekend begins this
evening and all I have to do is laundry, cleaning, grocery
shopping, seeing to the mowing of the grass, the tending of the
dogs, the changing of the litter boxes, the preparation of potato
salad and antipasto and the marinating of beef for shish kebab
for the family picnic. Like Scarlet O'Hara, however, I'll think

about all that tomorrow because it's entirely too beautiful a
night to worry about anything.

The last vestiges of a glorious May sundown are leaving
the sky and the dark and the cool are coming on fast. A dove
mourns nearby. An ultralight airplane, in gypsy colors, treadles
overhead like a sewing machine. Birds bicker about property
lines and such. A small white motorcycle purrs past. A birch
twig flexes a few leaves—not enough to rustle however. An
ancient lilac blooms as if she fears this might be her last season.
Just the faintest trace of a skunk wafts past.

Most of the unfenced yards nearby have already been
mowed for the big holiday weekend. We have *yards* here—
front yards, back yards, side yards, barn yards. Suburbs have
lawns but we have yards—except, of course, for the occasional
manicured, showered-and-shaved, footbound showplace
presided over, perhaps, by some compulsive soul. We have
green and growing and decently groomed, but not necessarily
grass. Friendly neighborhood trees drip blossoms—cherry,
plum, crabapple, 'thorne apple, flowering quince. Dandelions
are taking their stand and the maple trees, like flower girls at
a wedding, strew the driveway with seed helicopters.

Tuesday, June 25, 1984 — 6:17 a.m.

A film of night slumps over the trees now fat with leaf. A
moderate bird hops along the embedded stones, looking as if
he's misplaced his clipboard.

I'll be glad when the pins, which protrude from the tips
of my toes like five tiny Allen wrenches to immobilize them so
they can heal, can be removed and I can take a shower without
encasing my foot in garbage bags and freezer tape to prevent
water-borne infection. It's all so cumbersome, what with the
elaborate showering routines, the orthotic shoe with its flat
wooden sole that makes me walk like Frankenstein's monster,

sutures like razor wire threading through my toes. Even the description of the procedure is clumsy: metatarsal resection, partial phalangectomy of four toes, bunionectomy. But the pain is much reduced and—surprise!—my foot is quite a bit shorter than the other. The surgeon decided not to implant plastic joints in my toes because the bones were too deteriorated.

1 p.m.

While the birch tree trails its fingers possessively through my hair, the sun, just another high bright cloud, catches a roundish yellow butterfly and a husky thistle stalk rehearsing a *pas de deux*. A shimmer hovers etheric over the hot blacktop as a bold breeze warps the browning grass which covers the napping earth.

After 6 p.m.

Although I can still hear the relentless hum of the collective machine in the far distance, crickets preside now. Browning onions and charcoal starter scent the evening as cars crunch home on gravel driveways or back busily out for the evening. A few belligerent boys in ATVs are ripping up a nearby field.

Now the earth is up again and awake but quiet, perhaps will take tea and toast and enjoy the twilight and the cooler, drier air that has slipped in unannounced. But, no, forget that…Two lawn mowers have been fired up, and a battered black and brown motorcycle, looking as if it were made of flattened tin cans and buried in the sands of Iwo Jima since 1945, screams desperately past, trying to achieve second gear.

Tuesday, July 24, 1984

San Ysidro Massacre

At last homicidal, he slips the traces of humanity
under heavy arms he speeds
bloody justice
to those who'd had their chances
in the abscesses of his lost mind,
finds judgment
in his own splattered guts.

We have nothing to dilute our grief, we are
shocked that civilization
is a long, long series of choices.

Friday, August 3, 1984

My hands, my fingers
gnarled, faceless scrubwomen eyes
downcast, overshrouded by kneeling
skirts and babushkas, like grayed flannel drawsheets
tied at the napes,
scrub, scrub
yearn, yearn.

My hands, my fingers, necks
arched like show ponies, figure
skaters pumping into other dimensions
defy the law of averages
tune out the siren songs of history.

My carved feet, bulbous
in gauze turbans, levitate
at the ends of prickly legs
like works of surgical art.

Two down and two to go. My left foot has been carved
up to match my right—round two of swelling, orthotic shoe,
bandages, sutures, pins, post-surgical pain. For the first several
days afterwards, surgical trauma produces enough endorphins
to preclude the need for pain killers. But after that period, the
pangs of healing join forces with everyday RA pain and the
additional stiffness from decreased mobility. Managing all that
without more than aspirin is a true challenge. A worthwhile
challenge, nonetheless, because I'd prefer to not load my body
with any more chemicals and their effects than I've already
used. The anesthesia and tranquilizers and antibiotics and
topical antiseptics before, during, and immediately after the
surgeries, on top of the usual gold injections and twenty-four

aspirin daily, seem enough to ask a body to cope with. Meanwhile, I'm trying to maintain an appreciation of the long-term benefits of these surgeries as well as the short-term gains of this phase of my life, such as having time to soak up the beauty of our place and the seasons and to regain a measure of spiritual health.

I'm determined to use this interval between surgeries to regain some sort of psychological equilibrium. I've made arrangements to borrow whatever money I need to survive this period in some measure of comfort now that my source of income has dried up; I'll deal with repayment when I am again working. I've also scheduled several counseling sessions to help me find a healthier outlook than my usual one of abject terror.

Living near a country railroad accentuates all the romantic notions I've accumulated about trains—the plaintive mourning of the distant whistle in the late hours of night, the utter power of massive iron boxes rolling over glinting rails tied together by creosoted timbers. A bed of gravel and small white stones edges, like fancywork, the creek running shoulder-to-elbow with the railroad. Cattails, tiger lilies, brown-eyed Susans lounge nearby like so many prosperous farmers swapping crop talk at the Co-Op on a warm Saturday morning.

The children, in this last month of summer vacation, invite school friends to scuff the stones along the railroad and to poke among the rocky ruins of once-farmhouse cellars, to thrill to the discovery of a shard of green-tinted fruit jar, or a blue glass insulator from some bygone electrical connection. Sometimes they discover wild strawberries the size of early June peas and tracks—animal tracks!!!

Last fall a fawn prince mincing along the creek caught my scent and, by a brisk left flank maneuver and a ray of unblinking intelligence beaming through his wide black eyes

directly into mine, stopped me in my tracks as he bounded
away, it seemed, into the sky.

In the suburbs raccoons trespass trash containers and squat
in garage attics in early fall; here they are good neighbors—
provided allowances are made for them in the garden. Rabbits
populate every acre. Deer as regularly decimate corn crops as
skunks perforate the night in pursuit of the sickly white grubs
travelling incognito among the grass roots. Invisible moles
undermine the yard in pursuit of these same delicacies and
other subterranean morsels. Garter snakes and earthworms
can be found under any woodpile and rattlers sun themselves
on rocks in the field out back.

Monday, August 6, 1984

Overcast. Still. Silent. A brown rabbit flips his white undertail
backwards as he skitters through the brush across the road.
Invisible birds chatter. A dog yips.

> *Plain-speaking bumpkins*
> *en masse, fierce freckled menace*
> *bold tiger lilies.*

It has taken chronic illness and incapacitating surgery to
provide a block of time in which I can write every day but
this is only temporary; I still have to find my own way to do
what I wish to do, to earn a living by writing. Perhaps what
has been lacking is my decision, my real choice. Jung wrote,
"…unless one assents to the power of the inner voice, the
personality cannot evolve."

Tuesday, September 4, 1984

> *A hot apple falls*
> *lies light in state on soft grass*
> *the earth stops spinning.*

Today was Kevin's first day of high school. I truly can't
believe that he's fourteen already and Rain is twelve. The
time has passed entirely too quickly. There are so many things
I wanted to have done with them before they arrived at this
stage that will never be done now. All the more reason to
cherish the remaining years of their youth.

Saturday, September 29, 1984

Another family funeral—my youngest aunt, my namesake,
six years my senior, of myocardial infarction a few days *after*
bypass surgery.

Saturday, October 27, 1984 — 2:30 p.m.

With very shaky left hand, on day #11 after right hand surgery...
Another four hours in surgery and now I'm bionic,
according to my children. The joint capsules on the four
fingers of my right hand have been removed and Dow-
Corning joints have been countersunk in all the little bone
ends. With my right hand and arm swathed in bandages and
cradled in a splint, I watch hours and hours of television and
read reams and reams of printed material. But I miss writing
so I'm determined to learn to write well with my left hand.

Another of the mixed blessings of this surgical marathon
is having time and situation to evaluate my life. Unfortunately
I find less to congratulate than to correct.

I think these surgeries have followed too closely on each others' heels. I'm feeling spent and frail. I'm having sleep apnea, which is very frightening, and night sweats. To add insult to surgery, I've had a rash of obscene calls in the middle of the night. Per Michigan Bell's instruction, I'm keeping a log and, if the calls continue, Bell will monitor the line to see who's calling and prosecute.

Sunday, November 4, 1984

I've clipped a wonderfully encouraging article by Arianna Stassinopoulos, on Jonas Salk, that appeared in today's *Parade* Magazine. She writes,

> Jonas Salk likens conscious evolution to "a spreading infection, a veritable epidemic of integrity and responsibility with more and more people becoming carriers." He adds, "It is a law of nature, whether among human beings or among fruit flies, that evolutionary changes in behavior spread quickly through a built-in mechanism—as if there had been a town hall meeting or a report on the 7 o'clock news."

Stassinopoulos writes, "When we are preoccupied with survival, much of our behavior is dictated by fear—fear, as Jonas Salk has stressed time and again, that often has little to do with threats to our actual survival."

I know—I *know*—that it is *fear* that enabled this disease to take over my life. I've been aware that I've been motivated primarily by fear since as far back as I can remember. And according to the research cited in Kenneth R. Pelletier's *Mind As Healer, Mind As Slayer,* I am typical of women with RA.

I just finished reading Norman Cousins' *Anatomy Of An Illness* in which he designs a treatment plan for himself; I'd like to do likewise.

Sunday, January 27, 1985

After a week of melt-down and mud, these cusp mornings
are gray, melancholy, without promise or threat, unlike the
ominous gray days of November or the brooding calm of
tornado season. Disoriented by a sudden snow squall after
many days of spring, these days are stalled, neither fish nor
fowl.

The surgeries are finally finished. I'm exhausted and
oppressed by feelings of futility and defeat. Nothing would
suit me more than to stop where I am and never progress
another step. I feel like I'm home from the wars and I'd be
content to sit silently in an orchard and do nothing more than
smell apples. But I've been living on savings, credit, and the
kindness of friends for eight months and I must find another
job as soon as I can. Unfortunately, my hands won't be healed
enough and I won't look healthy enough to start interviewing
until perhaps early May.

I don't know how I could have gotten through these
surgeries without the help—housework, shopping,
chauffeuring, moral support, loans and cash—of friends and
family, especially my beautiful children.

Now my days are appointed by exercise sessions. I squeeze
rubber balls to regain flexibility in my right hand, and massage
my left to prevent adhesions. When my incisions are better
healed I'll learn to play a recorder as therapy for both hands.

Right now the thought of my customary work—
accounting—offers no reward but cash. I can't think that
my work adds anything to the world—not that I believe
that *anyone's* numbers or writing, the works of Shakespeare or
Michelangelo, or the seeing and saying of Dick and Jane and
Jesus *necessarily* have significance to anyone beyond their
creators. The real value is in the call, the desire to do and then
the doing, I think. There are prostitutes in every profession, I

know, who ply an art or craft for cash and not for love, but prostitution always destroys more than it supports, I think. Is it reasonable, at this eleventh hour, to think of starting over in any kind of work? Where am I headed?

> *If bonfires and ashes were again in vogue*
> *we'd smell again of smoke*
> *and make up stories*
> *of how we have the stars figured out.*

> *Go ahead. Pick your analogy*
> *your faith*
> *your hope and love*
> *your paradigm.*
> *Pay your money:*
> *Take your choice.*

> *I want to be the Italian grandfather*
> *all seven hills behind me looking out*
> *as the sun dances*
> *among the Romans below.*

Tuesday, February 5, 1985

Michigan Bell finally found the man who has been making the obscene calls and they are prosecuting even though the calls have stopped. I don't recognize his name so he must have picked my number from the telephone book. I'm going to change our number and not have our new number listed.

Thursday, April 4, 1985

Monday I'll be starting a new job at a company that fabricates machine tooling for the automotive industry. None of my

philosophical questions have been resolved by being hired
by this company but some *fiscal* ones certainly have been.

Saturday, July 6, 1985

Last summer I saw clouds of fireflies and hundreds of
dragonflies but this year I've seen only a few of each. Could
the reason be that last summer I divided my time between my
front porch and the orthopedic surgery department and this
year I spend eleven hours of every day in the care and feeding
of my job?

Three heavy motorcycles crawl majestically past and dry
old leaves rush giddily into their wake. The neighbor kids toss
lit jumping jacks into the street to twirl madly red, fire, green,
and—*ffft*—die. A hot breeze bearing a scent of water from
somewhere south of here mixes with the picnic revelry in
some nearby backyard.

Sunday, September 29, 1985

Lucy has breast cancer. She's undergoing chemotherapy and
there's every reason to be hopeful.

Sunday, November 3, 1985

Leafless sugar maple silhouettes, still as corpses, lean against the
morning sky and frosted brown leaves lie in state on still-lush
lawns. I crack the window and a peppery cold tingles my nose,
a chill starts in my shoulders and shudders downward. The
birds of summer seem still here and vocal. Frost melt sparkles
in the path of the sun.

Lucy and I talked for a long time last night after our
families had gone to bed. The chemotherapy has been awful

for her but her oncologist assures her that the radiation therapy to come will be much more bearable. I envy her strong faith which supports her so well now. I want to be closer to her again but we are both constrained by distance and our families and jobs. The telephone will have to do.

Sunday, December 8, 1985

"When you start abandoning your old beliefs or values, some very primal circuits get ignited. Before moving on, you have to clear away all your cherished beliefs," writes Marilyn Ferguson in *The Aquarian Conspiracy.*

Now is a good time to reassess. Kev is in high school and Rain will be next fall. Their father has married again. I am well enough employed at work for which I have a certain knack but not at work I dream about. Maybe I wouldn't like writing after doing it full-time but I can't just forget it without trying it. I would regret that.

Saturday, March 8, 1986 — 6 a.m.

A weaving, shifting tissue of moisture is being mopped around the turbulent gray atmosphere; invisible snow is already organizing into flat drifts sidewinding across the road. Brown leaves, like giant wheat flakes, windrow away from a gust then slither belligerently back toward their starting place.

The scummy remnants of a long and fierce winter have been dissipated by a two-week hiatus of spring-like weather, but I have yet to see an early bud. The birch and red maple that inhabit our front yard remain stolid, adamant in their winter substance; they may have loosened their mufflers but they were no more moved by the brief respite than they are now by this building storm.

A sheet of hail blows by and momentarily blurs the scene across the road. This hard, granular stuff is accumulating among the pebbles on the shoulders of the road and the rows of utility pole pines across the street are only dark gray shadows. The tattered bark of the red maple in the middleground and, in the foreground, an unkempt shrub with snippets of straw and bits of leaf in its hair, stand in sharp relief, in full color—like a Viewmaster slide.

The TV weatherman is talking about thirty-five-foot ice piles and water cresting at seven feet above flood stage, warning residents of the shorelines of Lake Erie and Lake St. Clair to move cars and valuables to higher ground.

5:30 p.m.

Aside from the flurries following a downdraft from the porch roof, now only the mist slants across the gray, outlining the cracks in the road and settling along the needles of the now-black shrub. Now the spots without bark on the red maple are raw wounds, the only color.

We spent the entire day doing warm chores—laundry, ironing, homework, cooking ahead for the week. I've always regretted that this house has no fireplace because this would be a perfect night to spend in front of a cozy fire.

Sunday, May 11, 1986 — Mothers' Day, 5:15 a.m.

If I dropped my assumption that I and my kind are the center of the universe, I might assume that birds are. Hundreds browse, promenade, skim, skirmish, and chatter all around me while only several of my kind appear in the few acres I can see.

My silent companion is an exhausted cat. She's had the benefit of a middle-class upbringing—shots, spaying, proper cat food, pretty elastic collar—yet she clings to her more primitive drive to hunt and mate at night, to sleep when day comes, to leave a hair-shadow wherever she chooses, to ignore us most of the time and still to offer us a model and symbol of natural life and its consequences—without our permission.

Saturday, May 17, 1986

I have a hunger to go on a camping retreat, if only in our back yard. I want to get outside walls and structures and routines and take in the words of some wise writers with nothing else man-made surrounding me. The part of me that waited motionless to be blessed by a rain shower advancing from across Lake Huron needs communication with the silence of a groundfire. Sometimes I think all truly significant communication is silent. Perhaps it would be worthwhile sometimes to eliminate all other and observe the results.

I hate losing touch with this little piece of land but it's so easy to slip into the attitude that the land, the earth, the outdoors, are negligible, mere grout in the mosaic of reality. The important pieces, we seem to believe, are the buildings, landscaped playgrounds and resorts and parks, the institutions, economic theories, and manufactured goods. Nature is seen as mere raw material awaiting transformation and the infusion of life and significance by the better ideas of man.

Once land is claimed it should be used, occupied, savored, and not merely owned and profited from. Its capacities to feed, to shelter, to teach should be exercised and appreciated. It's wrong to leave house and land and captive animals alone and unoccupied every day in order to travel to another place and return only to do the barest minimum and sleep the regulated sleep of the common person.

Today I'm settling for a walk in the muddy yard and reading on the porch. Kev is bussing tables at The Bone Yard until eleven and Rain is spending the night at Kara's so I have the time, the books, and the silence, if not the camp and the groundfire.

Your expressions become entrained
with a thought in my mind, that same word
has been breathed into both of us.

I want to stay in your company
you magnify me
I feel the gods closer.

Sometimes you speak in tongues
I don't understand
and I am glad to be alone.

Sometimes we share such harmonies
the gods must be trapped
between us.

...from *Waiting For God,* by Simone Weil: "It is God who seeks man....It does not rest with the soul to believe in the reality of God if God does not reveal this reality."

It is God who seeks man. What an amazing thought.

...from Henry David Thoreau: "There is no more fatal blunderer than he who consumes the greater part of his life getting a living."

Tuesday, June 10, 1986

I'm feeling much better. For months I've felt like Al Capp's cartoon character, Joe Btfsplk, whose personal black cloud followed him everywhere.

The sun peeks from its oblique attitude to backlight airborne dandelion fluff, a wasp, a cloud of gnats, and a dragonfly who will sew up my ears if I allow it to get too close. The wasp flies as if its hind parts don't want to come along.

A breeze from the blind side of the house is fresh and sweet as it streams past the open windows but the rooms are still and stale and humid. Shadows spread themselves across the yard like cool sheets on a bed thrown wide and welcoming. Most of the trees are in full summer dress already. Japanese maples and Crimson Kings are the redheads of treedom, Russian olives the graying gentry. Sunburst Locusts are strictly punk.

Six or eight species of birds avail themselves of the lawn smorgasbord of bugs and worms and seeds. Birds could make do with only one leg since they seem only to hop anyway. Birds rarely left-right-left walk—except penguins, of course. Nature is more redundant than efficient.

The day promises to be hot but right now it's a perfect 75°, with a steady little breath from the southwest.

I do love this place. If I were completely alone I might hug this steady birch that has withstood so many ice storms that held her bent backwards for days at a time. I might again lay full-length, face-down to taste the soil, its heat and green. I might lay on my back and allow insects to crawl inside my clothing, grass to itch my skin, to contemplate the sky, the vast sky, the planet so immense I can't begin to sense its roundness.

I was born upon this planet in such a season; I'm freshened by its return. Sometimes I think that if I spend too much time outdoors, I'll never go back indoors again. My housekeeping will become ever more primitive and I'll become ever more feral. Then I'll die alone, disreputable, penniless and content.

Wednesday, December 17, 1986

Lucy died of breast cancer. Where there was hatred, she sowed love. Where there was injury, she sowed pardon. Where there was doubt, she sowed faith. Where there was despair, she sowed hope. Where there was darkness, she sowed light. Where there was sadness, she sowed joy.

Friday, February 27, 1987

The bright sky is cloud-mottled and such fresh air has not passed through these parts for a year. Scabs of grimy snow heal into dust along the curbs and the last of the clean snow fades into the restless brown grass. This ragged glory can't be appreciated by those who have wintered in places south; only those who have stood by our winded frozen land can finally value the sweet kiss of a February sun.

The track team is already in training and all of Rain's once-vibrantly-colored running clothes are a permanent mud-brown. I envy her running.

My RA is much worse in my head, hands, feet, shoulders. The gold therapy just isn't working at all any more even though I'm back to weekly injections. I'm sick of weekly blood drawing, urinalysis, and injections; I hate taking so many aspirin every day.

Saturday, July 4, 1987 — Independence Day

The sun is still lying on its side on the horizon and beaming through all the bearded dandelions. Brighton Lake is greeting-card blue and stippled with white as the last of the mists of the night fades into the warming morning. A vendor unlocks his paddle boats and drags the chains noisily up the dock. A truck tools along the gravel service road, emptying trash bins and shagging litter. A man with a green hose and a jug of bleach heads toward the cinderblock washrooms. An elderly couple across the roped-off swimming bay has chosen a table nestled in a birch grove and, although I can't see it, steam must be rising from the Thermos container they just opened; I can smell the coffee from here.

If all goes as I hope, I'll be able to spend a great part of today doing my two favorite things, writing and eating. The kids and I have come early to reserve enough tables for a reunion pot-luck of this generation of our branch of the family and everyone else will be along in an hour or two. Rain and Kev are still doing the heavy lifting, carrying the coolers, chairs, and food cross-country from our car while I guard our stake.

Surgery turned out to be a key element in my finally believing in my responsibility for my own life and health. Surgery was always my ace in the hole if the disease stayed active; and I'd heard I could have surgery as often as needed. I'd seen TV programs on the technology and the state of the arts of joint replacement and anesthesiology and it all seemed so locked in and nailed down.

I did all the homework I could think to assign myself and then agreed to a series of four surgical procedures beginning in the summer of 1984, which kept me anesthetized for more than six hours each time, over a period of eight months. I made myself an enlightened consumer, a careful and attentive patient, and I relaxed into confidence of success and considerable restoration despite the fact that I knew surgery couldn't arrest underlying disease.

Tuesday, September 1, 1987 — Mother's funeral

As if some mold has finally been broken, we were unable to have Mom's wake at Cliff Read's where all four of our grandparents, six uncles, four aunts, our dad, our brother Roger, and our sister Kathy were laid out over the years. Cliff Read died years ago and the business is now called the Read-Schultz Funeral Home. Read-Schultz had no space available so we had to use Clyne's, the protestant funeral home in Roseville, and the people there were most kind and accommodating.

We were unable to conveniently arrange a requiem mass at St. Barnabas Church but Mom probably wouldn't have cared anyway because, despite all the shock, anger, and despair for my immortal soul when I was married in a Unitarian church in 1968, she too had eventually thought her way out of the church.

For old times sake, we did say the rosary the first night of her wake, and one of my classmates, who was still in the priesthood, led prayers at the grave site next to Daddy's grave in Sacred Heart Cemetery. Her pall bearers were four of her six sons and two of her four daughters. She lived beyond her seventieth birthday, a record in her family.

Tuesday, September 8, 1987

Nearly five weeks since I've had a gold injection. I had to stop the injections again because I again developed mouth ulcers but, oddly, I've been a little better since I stopped the gold.

For more than a year, this area has been spooked by the elusive "Wixom Panther," said to be responsible for the demise of several goats and sheep and reported to have been sighted by a number of people in various neighborhoods. We worried about our two black Labs, afraid that perhaps the panther might leap over the fence into the yard and attack one of the dogs.

Last night, Blackie, the more brazen of our dogs, jumped the fence herself and headed into the woods. Hours later and worried sick, we watched her jump back in, safe and sound. I wonder how many times she was "sighted"...

Sunday, October 4, 1987

When I was awakened just after sunrise by the whoosh of the burners of three hot air balloons passing over the house, the earth was still snuggled under a sheet of fine frost, a puffy fog blanket beneath a shyly smiling sky. Now, in the sweet breeze of afternoon, the balance of the birch leaves leap to their rest in the waiting grass below as the day warms to perfect Indian Summer and curly, crunchy red and russet leaves migrate to evergreen hammocks and kumquats do one-armed push-ups on their leafless branches.

Thursday, October 22, 1987

I've found a rheumatologist whose office is closer to work so I can schedule appointments on my lunch hours. My supervisor is disgruntled that I've had to take time off work every week to see my doctor.

My knees were unbearably inflamed and painful so this new doctor recommended aspiration of the fluid from the joints and an injection of cortisone. I've heard so many horror stories about cortisone that I was reluctant to agree to this, but the doctor assured me that these stories refer to cortisone taken by mouth. He says that steroids injected into a joint have an entirely different action in the body and don't cause the adverse reactions that are caused by oral steroids. I hope he's right.

Friday, October 23, 1987 — 5:30 a.m.

Wow! This stuff is miraculous! I can't believe I feel so well and can move so freely! I have no pain and no stiffness. I am utterly comfortable! A slight jitteriness is the only negative thing I'm feeling. I can't wait for the kids to get up and find me *not* huddled in my chair waiting for aspirin to thaw out my stiff joints!

Friday, October 30, 1987

The cortisone is still working! I've been making up for lost time by blitzing our poor neglected house with soap and mops. I can even go into the basement with relative ease. I carved a jack-o-lantern this evening—the first one in many years.

One bad thing I've noticed since I had the cortisone injection is how quickly I can slip into a despondent mood; combined with my elation about being so mobile, I've become almost manic-depressive. And I have the most dreadful dreams; I feel that I'm dying as I try to slip off into sleep.

Tuesday, November 17, 1987

Windy tonight. Leaves tumble across the open fields and plaster themselves against fences and rustle into corners as the wind whistles through windows not locked up tight.

I had my knee aspirated again and another cortisone injection. The effects of the first injection lasted about three weeks altogether, but they began diminishing about six or seven days after the injection and gradually wore off. I've been getting progressively worse for the last week or so. I'm not going to make a habit of these injections so I hope the oral gold, Auranofin, I'm now taking will be more effective than the injected form.

The cat from hell, Duran, the newest baby in our house, springs to the back of my chair, softly brushes my neck, and descends my left arm to rest, purring loudly, on my notebook. She lays her head back to afford me the opportunity to stroke her silky throat then begins to knead my thigh. She bumps her ear against my idle hand until I scratch it then abruptly drops to the floor to saunter to her dish. She pursues her own life, not a cat's life or a life like that of Licorice, our senior cat. I think cats are a teaching device employed by an easy-going god and all living is a story problem.

Friday, November 27, 1987

Your tracks are everywhere
fresh forever
like light
in a closed mirror-system.

A cold rain has been falling steadily for over twelve hours. I don't want to discount this season of dormancy and the return of waters expended but I must also bear in mind and trust that spring will follow and a summer of new life, figurative as well as literal.

Until I was twenty I saw my happiness and salvation within the peaceful walls of the convent where life was ordered and secure, decisions were made by superiors, and God provided unbroken serenity. After I discovered the chips and cracks in the walls of the convent, I sought fulfillment in a season of political and religious activism, hoping to somehow find peace in chaos, order in anarchy, and God in no conviction at all. Later it became obvious to me that society was right and my hope must be in a man and marriage and children. Now I see that happiness is self-generated from nothing at all and life is an art object created as any painting or sculpture is created—not photographically obedient to some diagram like a middle school shop project, and not primarily from experience, but as inspired by the soul.

Now I see the soul as a piece of God, an unseverable umbilical cord between God and the universe, the chip on which resides all of history, the germ of all wisdom and all power, life itself. Its tools are the mind, the brain, the body, the cosmos. The soul is the parent while the mind, brain, and body are the offspring.

Sunday, November 29, 1987

The morning is packed in fog and silence. Winter has still not come yet, but spring temperatures and rain rush premature into the void.

Cortisone day #11. The effect is already reduced by about half.

Tuesday, December 1, 1987

The many faces of the first snow of 1987:

Out the back windows, gaunt black maples doze in white wooly mantles and warm brown weeds lay down on their sides. The sticking snow has lulled the land to sleep, hibernating into the accumulated gray and promise of snows to come. Rest. Peace.

In lamp glow, the Christmas card view through the front window features broad white snow planes atop story-book houses with cozy gold windows and curly gray smoke. Furry shrubs, backsides free of snow, like boys who've forgotten to brush the hair on the backs of their heads, wait at the edges of the porch for the storms and drifts to come. Promise, adventure.

In town, through falling snow, the houses across the lake and the cars on the misty road drift delicately atop stilts of light in melted snow. The road hisses and absorbs the wisps of steam escaping tailpipes. Mystery. Romance.

Is love of freedom an acquired taste? Many people I know seem to feel no discomfort within the various harnesses and fences fashioned by society and imagined to be from the gods, but I always have. One of my most frightening and empathic moments was watching Kunta Kinte struggle against a neck iron in the television production of Alex Haley's *Roots*. I can visualize myself, in such a situation, going wild and unravelling mentally, my heart and lungs and gut bursting from rage, my springs unwinding into a berserk heap of ravaged life.

Warring with society, chauvinism, materialism, withholding are activities that do more violence to me than to my opponents. Tailgaters will kill me yet, unless I learn to live in peace with them.

Tailgaters are the bane of my driving existence. When one appears in my rear-view mirror, I hope that the body English of my anxious and exaggerated glances into the rear-view mirror will alone remind the driver to ease off to make a safer space between our vehicles. If that fails, I gradually slow down then quickly speed up to create that safe space myself. If that doesn't work, I slow considerably and tap the brake repeatedly to blink my brake lights to suggest a need for caution and distance. Most times, I end up pulling over onto the shoulder to allow the offender to pass, often shaking and shouting obscenities, while I am faint, red-faced, palpitating, and murderous. My punishment has indeed hurt me more than it hurt the other.

Why does a driver tailgate? Arrogance? Aggressiveness? Ignorance? Poor judgment? Poor memory? Poor depth perception? Inattention? Distraction? What does it matter? The fact is still that he is tailgating.

All things considered, the best solution is to learn to ignore the pressures of others and refuse to cave in to them. To move out of the way of the tailgater is to solve the problem of the moment yet perhaps to create a new problem. Re-entry into traffic might be very difficult, the next driver behind might be another tailgater—or a drunk—and the offending behavior is reinforced. The best solution is to focus on my own goals with respectful consideration and appropriate accommodation of reasonable others. If I ignore his bullying unreasonable demand, will the tailgater sooner or later alter his behavior? Will he notice, pay attention, learn, change, acquiesce, or remember if tailgating nets him nothing—or if he crashes into me? Living is choice, isn't it? But I can't change anything but myself.

Thursday, December 3, 1987

Yesterday's wet snow shower continued gently throughout most of the day. Now the shrubs, swollen and billowing, slouch heavily against the house and over the rail fence across the street as cars swish softly by on the salted street.

Saturday, December 5, 1987

One boneless cat oozes over the sofa back she straddles and studies the uneaten crusts of Thursday's snow; another lies curled like a furry larva in a sunpatch.

Today's sun is brilliant as summer. Icicle-drip waters the bedraggled porch bushes still clumped with snow.

An old dream visits me again. I'm thirteen and my right shoe hits the porch, my left the second step, and I'm off like a shot across the gravel driveway, across Ten Mile Road, barely checking for traffic. My foot hits the gray sidewalk and I churn past Moody's. Over the cracked walk, I speed past weed fields and Cope's house, Berendts' store, Ed's barber shop, fields of clover and Queen Anne's lace, past Woody's drive filled with Harley-Davidsons. I pump harder past Brown's dairy, Leises' store. I pass McSwain's restaurant, with a faded CLOSED sign in its grubby front window draped in cobweb. I've hit my stride and I'm only skimming now. Now my feet never touch the ground as I streak past a row of sprawling brick bungalows with wide gracious roofs and broad front porches, past horse chestnut trees and lilac bushes that overhang the walk. Past Memorial field I don't feel the ground beneath my feet.

Another block blurs beneath me, then another. I speed up, pace myself to allow a car to pass, then diagonally re-cross Ten Mile Road and turn right onto Dodge Street. Pass Fishers'— no kids in the yard—and stop at Manchester.

I turn right and regulate my breath and knock brightly on a wooden screen door. Grandma Nies, smelling of Sweetheart soap and Tabu perfume, beams and fusses and gives me cantaloupe with vanilla ice cream in her cool kitchen.

Tuesday, February 2, 1988

> *I am failed again*
> *of all those foreign goals and standards*
> *to which I have hauled myself up again*
> *to make up in volume again*
> *what was lacked in substance. I must bear*
> *in mind: these are not my gods.*

Forehead against the cold glass, I'm surprised by the puffs of airy new snow perching on every branch, a three-inch blanket comforting the car in the drive. A soft blue nightlight still glows amid the skeletons of black trees, the morning star, an invisible moon, a sun beyond the curve of the planet.

Away from the windows, the lamp blackens the glass and reflects only what is inside, as if to void any reality outside this cold house, and renders this box of light and the whir of the furnace all the more cozy and comforting.

I dress hastily and I'm off, coffee mug in mittened hand. Viewing this luminous moment through glass is not enough; neither is gaping from the porch while the astringent air shrinks the lining of my nose.

No, I must tramp through this snow and examine the accumulation on every shrub. I must inspect up close its effect on last summer's worm-bags, still clutching at the crotches of the crabapple tree. I must try to see the entire effect of the winter on the vacant squirrel nest high in the red maple. I must look at the night's tracks in the new snow. I must let this blue glow work its magic on me.

7:30 p.m.

Alas, I did my duty. I performed my usual ablutions, donned my usual work uniform, drank the afore-mentioned coffee, and spent more than eight hours accounting for the dollars of someone I don't know, doing business I neither respect nor admire, without pleasure and only for dollars of my own.

My day was spent in a windowless box of synthetic materials among robots of the electronic and human varieties. According to the plan, I will do likewise tomorrow. And the following day. And the next. Until age sixty-five, broken only at weekly intervals to allow time to acquire more stuff, to consume great quantities of potables, amusements, and to display my accumulation.

I imagine Venus still where she was in the southeastern sky twelve hours ago. The night is opaque black and bluntly, windlessly cold. With no wind, these latitudes nap until moonrise. Perhaps the sun shone today and the air warmed and compacted the morning's fluffy snow into the dense quilt now comforting the shrubs near the porch. I don't know; I wasn't here.

I think the original sin was the abandonment of living directly on the surface of the earth and no longer sustaining life directly from the gifts of earth. By this choice of indirect living, humanity sold itself into slavery to the less-than-genius schemes of all the organizers of the earth.

Friday, February 5, 1988

A grapefruit-colored blaze ignites the horizon and x-rays the atmosphere, projecting exaggerated shadows across the snow. Night swept the loose surface into erratic windrows, exposing brown grass spikes and tumbling winter's windfalls into heaps against the fence. Sunny as it is, a fine powder drives, almost invisible, on a sturdy wind.

This is the season for appreciating the internal workings of the planet, the parts that abide after the flowering and the fruiting, the glory and demise of its days in the sun. This is the season to appreciate the contemplative dormant phase that follows a season in the fields. I and the planet are at home to lie fallow until the sap again begins to rise.

Saturday, February 7, 1988

In the grocery store this morning, a little boy, maybe four years old, spent a long time studying my hands and finally asked, "Hey, what's wrong with your hands?" I liked his direct approach a lot better than the surreptitious glances I usually get from adults, from whose painful courtesy I'd like to deliver them. It was easy for me to explain to that little boy that I have a disease and that I've had surgery to repair some of the damage as well as to replace my diseased joints with plastic ones, and that although my hands look funny they work really well and I like them a lot. His response was a simple, "Oh."

I wish people would ask more often, if they're curious, because I wonder what strange conclusions they might otherwise draw. I know that I'm usually mistaken when without checking facts I draw conclusions instead of merely expressing observations or, at most, hunches or working theories.

Monday, February 9, 1988

This disease that racks my footsteps
ties my hands bares
my soft pink underbelly disarms
my foes I surrender.
I survive.

I might have chosen to do battle and died, dying
not knowing
is worse.

Impaled upon a webwork of birch shoots high in the southern sky, the moon highlights a brittle stillness. Yesterday's high winds and snow devils have left a sensation of respite in their wake. I catch my breath and slide the fogged glass, closing out the overwhelming cold.

I have a constant need to recalibrate, to touch solid ground after time spent in the clouds, to see the sun after times in the depths of the mines, to rest on the seventh day. I've seen nature as a haven, a retreat, a return to the womb more often than I've viewed it as a goal, a promised land, a never-never land, a land of milk and honey. I've been unable to think of enrichment as long as I've felt pain.

Perhaps escape and pain relief *are* to be found on the journey to the stars—but surely they are lesser milestones. I want to move far beyond merely surviving a disease and a system. I want to discover and fulfill the *real* purpose of life.

Some say the way to discover truth is to create it, to imagine it and believe it. Perhaps it's necessary only to *declare* it.

Wednesday, February 11, 1988

A sabbath of sorts, no new snow fell last night after six straight nightfalls. Yesterday's afternoon sun melted enough snow to create pencil-size icicles along the south edge of the roof. The accumulated snow is deflated and dense, stolid, settled in for the duration.

Thursday, February 12, 1988

Granular snow drops, vertical and ernest, through the windless air and piles yet another layer on the accumulation of so many days. Except for a few porch lights, there is no visible source of the dull pinkish glow squatting on the southern horizon—the city, I guess. At the back of the house, to the north, a vapor of

light seems to be rising through a navy sky. There may be a
moon and a million stars overhead—or a star and a billion
moons—but I can't know; I'm in my box.

Saturday, February 14, 1988

The neighbors' black pine hangs plumb and heavy from the
hook of the thick rind of the moon. Futuristic, other-worldly
snow sculptures, blown in on the night's winds, have displaced
the pristine expanse of ten inches of new snow which fell
yesterday. Slashed by four-foot drifts, three-foot snow walls line
the chute our driveway has become. Every bough is frosted
thick. The atmosphere is black but clear; visibility must be a
hundred miles. Nothing moves now but I hear the wind
having the last word.

My knees and shoulders are really bad this morning. The
weekly injections don't seem to be helping. I'll be glad when
we finish all the chores on the list today. We have to get salt
for the water softener, straw for the dogs, and feed for all the
animals at the co-op; the usual groceries, plus we must make
stops at the library, the bank, and the post office. Both kids
are scheduled to work this afternoon.

I soaked some white beans last night and started baking
them, with molasses, bacon, and onion, at six when I got up.
They're starting to smell good already and they should be done
when we get back. I'll make some muffins to go with them,
and maybe coleslaw.

Monday, February 23, 1988

In 1975 I began writing poetry and stories and letters and
a journal and aphorisms and jokes and essays and sermons.
I felt as though I were undergoing meltdown. Divorced and

imploding in 1978, I realized I wanted to write for a living. I've thought about it, planned, speculated, talked and obsessed about the idea every day since.

I did write. I submitted some things for publication and one magazine publisher actually accepted two short stories and five poems. I was so excited when I got the letter and the legal forms and a request for a brief writing bio! But the magazine folded before my writing saw print. After that, my publishing efforts went dormant but I wrote relentlessly on. Then my quill was always dipped in body fluids; now I mostly write with scratchy rock shards on chipped slate with waxy patches.

Every night I promise myself I will write something creative the next day, regardless of how I feel, but I'm doing well if I actually manage to make a few notes in this journal.

Saturday, April 2, 1988

> *She wakens early to tapping*
> *overhead new warmth upon the wind*
> *stands docile*
> *long-grown hair streaming*
> *her back drenched*
> *in spring*
> *deliverance.*

I'm feeling better these past weeks. Maybe the weekly injections are finally helping. Maybe the music of the frogs in the marshes around here has triggered some healing reflex in me. Maybe the buds on the trees have reminded my body that it knows how to heal itself. Maybe the wizened old lilac in the backyard, pushing out graceful sprays of lavender flowers, has shamed my younger limbs into trying harder.

I saw a lone brave wild strawberry blossom just outside the mown edge of our yard. The field beyond is still pretty wet but maybe I'll take a walk out there this afternoon to see what else believes that spring is truly here.

Sunday, May 15, 1988

On Thursday the second, barefoot, in shorts and tee-shirt, with a plate of Campbell's Scotch Broth in my hand, rushing to answer the telephone, I lost my balance, spilled the soup, slipped in it, fell, and was stunned by hitting my head on the leg of the kitchen table. I couldn't get up and was alone in the house and all the doors were locked. I dragged myself on a lubricant of soup to the telephone and called Kev who was at Bob's house, five miles away. Fortunately, he was there, he had keys, and he had a car.

When Kev tried to pick me up I became certain something was broken so I lay there among the vegetables while he called EMS. My right knee was as big as a cantaloupe. An ambulance came, and a fire truck, and the neighbors watched from their driveways. We crawled through rush hour traffic to the hospital where Kev had been born nearly eighteen years ago.

The emergency room was temporarily closed after we arrived because of a deluge of crash victims from a freeway pile-up. The triage nurse didn't put me at the top of her list. We waited.

My knee grew to the size of a baby watermelon as I lie there on a gurney wearing vegetables. Kev called his dad who rushed over with Rain. We all waited and Rain picked food out of my hair. After all the bleeding people had been attended to—no one was seriously injured—my turn came.

Fractured pelvis. Dislocated knee. Soft cast on my leg. Time will mend the fracture. Acetaminophen with codeine will help with the pain. I took it. It helped. But I still hurt like hell for about a week.

My Great Soup Caper took the edge off of the joy of Kev's acceptance at the University of Wisconsin and Rain's championship track season.

Monday, June 27, 1988

I wrote a check to the ambulance company for $260. For some reason I was under the impression that such emergency services are paid for by the city or the county. Surprise, surprise!

Kev has been graduated with honors from high school and is almost out the door to college. He's flipping hamburgers for the summer and Rain has a job at a boutique selling pewter and lead crystal. They're grown up; I can't believe it.

Here we go again. My heart is breaking. I'm going to have to sell the house and soon. With Kev going off to college, and my health being so unpredictable, Rain and I need to be in a place where we don't have almost an acre of grass to mow and the leaves of twenty mature trees to rake.

I'm going to miss being here. We've had the best of both worlds with a place in the country near enough a freeway to have the best parts of the city.

Tuesday, August 2, 1988

I hate leaving the house and the children to go to work, especially this last summer of this phase of our lives together and these last months in this house. I wish we could spend this last month without jobs or other obligations. But, alas, we do have jobs, Kev has preparations to make for college, Rain runs daily with the cross country team, and they both spend evenings and weekends with friends, and daily hours on the telephone.

Am I just sad because the children are moving ever closer to the edge of the nest, or because I am so disheartened by everything I hear on the news? Both? Both.

The details of the news never change so why do I bother watching and reading the news? It's a habit. I'm stuck in the same way civilization is stuck. Society has been stalled at this level because it was the *first* stage of effective control which felt like the *final* stage, home; we just stopped looking. Took the first answers that seemed to work. Like war, classes, hierarchies, materialism. Now we live too far off the land and our over-choice is blinding and crippling.

We're blinded by the appetites of our bodies and by the prevailing notion that we're no more than our bodies and brains—and our stuff. Our bodies, our newest, most fragile and temporary parts, seem most *us* because of size and their ability to detect each other and other things on the planet.

Yet I believe each person knows inside herself that the *essential she* exists permanently with or without intake and output devices, like the five popular senses and memory, hands, feet, and hormones. And I believe that unexamined thought is so frightening that we try to drown it with ever more activity and ever more stuff.

Friday, August 5, 1988, 6:15 a.m.

Michigan is having a record-hot, drought-dry summer. Yesterday the air temperature reached 100° and the heat index of 113°. All evening I was drenched and exhausted, breathing heavily because of high ozone levels and high humidity in the atmosphere.

I awakened this morning to the same heat, the same humidity, the same stagnant air and odors, the same dread of trying to pull on clothing over un-dryable skin, the same loginess. The hall thermometer seems welded at 80°.

I opened the door to let in Licorice, our stalker-of-nights, and she herself was being shadowed by a thick fog ribbon laying in wait across the road. The outside air was still heavy with the odors of many days—but at least the porch thermometer showed a cool 75°! The moral of the story: one must seek fame, fortune, and comfort outside the familiar— or at least see what the cat drags in!

Two ladies slowly pedal their coaster bikes back and forth on our mile of road. The neighborhood teems with blackbirds and but only the occasional car passes by. Coffee and toast ride the airwaves. An invisible trash truck labors audibly. Faint evidence hangs in the thinning fog that Mr. Skunk was here again during the night. Duran, our Darling Cat, pursues a moth into a shrub and it's so quiet I can hear her footfall on the orange needles on the earth below.

6:30 p.m.

A woman in my position could cause a garter snake
to thistle away or comment on the string art of guy
wires propping TV transmissions and pinkly
winking at a flashing metal insect
monitoring the dying day.

From this viewpoint a woman could spy
on aluminum dragonflies crouched over chimneys stalking
children's ears to sew or
hear a stony brook doing its Tennyson thing
and smell a cedar thicket making peat.

I, a sleeping Amazon—well, dreaming anyway
might trace a ring of dry worm dung or roll
over and spit a stiff
ant into a blue shell fragment
or the nest overhead
stupidly dangling sidewise, like a G.I. Christmas ornament,
by a length of bald yarn.

Tuesday, September 20, 1988

My house is an egg, an incubator, warmed by my furnace, bright by my lamps, quiet by my insulation, isolated by my walls. I open the door and find the world cooler, busier, darker. Inside I manage to maintain a year-round 72°, but outside the cosmos forces its cycles and preferences upon me. I understand it is I who must make peace with creation and not the other way around.

I'm grieving the absence of my firstborn who lives now in a dorm four hundred miles from here. The three months until he returns for Christmas break will last years. My younger child, my baby, now sixteen, is strengthening her own wings as she runs the roads with the cross-country team each day and exercises her twenty-day-old license to drive. In two years she too will drop below my horizon.

My RA has been less than stable for some time now. Gold salts injections every week, twenty-four aspirin daily, and occasional steroid injections limit its progress to a crawl but still the deterioration and deformity continue. Only the pain and stiffness are consistent.

I'm bitter even though I do *try* to be philosophical about my growing loss. I know how silly it would be to ask "why me?" Why anyone? Why any disease? But these aren't even genuine rhetorical questions because I realize that such things are impersonal parts of the evolutionary process. Still…

I tolerate my RA; I co-exist with it, knowing which of us has the upper hand. But I still can't believe that the only available treatments are those sanctioned by the Arthritis Foundation. Recently I learned that there is an organization that maintains a data base of information on folk medicine and other ways of treating diseases but I haven't been able to locate a name so far. It's as if there's an information underground and I can't seem to locate its entry or I don't have enough time to look for it.

Thursday, November 10, 1988

We're almost packed to move, the brothers have been lined up, the deposit has been paid on the rental truck, the cleaning is almost finished. The riffling winds of change have become gales as the pages of our history turn again.

Each time I board up windows, batten hatches, bring the children in. I secure what I can and shelter what can't be nailed down. We've been through these storms before and each time we've managed to rebuild in our own image and likeness.

Saturday, December 10, 1988

Here in Walled Lake there's a legend that many moons ago there were two warring Indian tribes which each claimed the lake as its own. They resolved the problem, the legend says, by dividing the lake into two parts with a brick wall built across the lake bed below the surface of the water.

I wonder what the Potawatomi Indians, who lived in these parts for many years, might have thought about this story if they'd heard it, since I know that Indians do not believe in the ownership of parts of Mother Earth. They believe that people belong to Earth rather than the other way around.

The house in Wixom belongs now to a nice young family and Rain and I have moved five miles up the road to a condo in Walled Lake. The red maples and the birch and the blue spruce and the fields and the critters, wild and domestic, didn't move with us.

Tup the bunny (who began her life with us as Buttercup and became Cuppie, Tuppie, Tupperware, Tup) has returned to Sunshine Farm, from whence she came. Charlie, the garter snake, long ago made a break for freedom under the garage in Westland and the lizards, Starbuck and Slippy, disappeared inside the house there. The fish that ate the other fish were given to neighbor friends.

After six months of TLC, Bbugg still hadn't recovered enough to leave her box when she began having seizures again; she died soon afterwards. Good Sam, whom we adopted when the people two houses down moved and abandoned him in the dead of winter, had died of feline leukemia, which he already had, I realize now, when we took him in. We worked for more then six months to find a home for our pair of eight-year-old, rowdy, sixty-pound lovable dogs. Duran moved to Bob's, and Licorice moved with us.

A tag hanging around the neck of the glorious red poinsettias presiding over our dining area says that poinsettias were merely straggly weeds that happened to be red at Christmas time until someone got the bright idea to use them as Christmas flowers. Since then they have been studied, curried and combed, and super-bred to produce the robust beauties we all know and love. No one pulls them out by the root anymore and no one talks herbicide. We should note that dandelions occur with the return of spring...

Monday, February 6, 1989 — looking at the 6 a.m. sky

Here in the city, the horizon is a roofline, and the panoramic view is concrete, cars, and stilted vegetation. Daylight itself is sucked up by the blacktop and parched aluminum. Nothing is returned to the earth or the atmosphere. Life is not inert here—it is nearly dead. Here one looks upward or one falls into a deep, stark sleep.

I reach for the sky for perspective, for a unifying principle. I imagine a panoramic Indian sky of the southwest—broad and blue. Or a cathedral sky arching over a forest of towering pines. Or a starry, starry night sky. Even a gray neighborhood sky will do to put the things in my mind in better relationship with the things in my soul.

At any hour of any day, the sky puts me back in conscious touch with my nature, with the cosmos, with my search for God. I can't stand conscious under any sky and feel separate from or superior to any other aspect of creation—attitudes all too easy to maintain inside a low-ceilinged office or store, a shadowy boudoir, or any church with spires no higher than the ladders of man. All worship should be under the open sky, where self-congratulation is clearly lit, so Truth alone will be adored.

I want to change my work—but how? My voices—my angels and my demons both—tell me to simply express my thought in writing, not for the enlightenment of others but for their observation if they wish. They remind me, frighten me, that my expression carries no merit, is key to no other life. They insist that writing is simply what *I* should do to wait comfortably for God.

I want to change my life, to create something. To actually *add* something without subtracting anything. Yet life is constantly consuming other life. My flesh-eating is covered by a pall of immorality and even vegetarianism, like our creation of God, is anthropomorphic; we don't eat what bleeds like us, or has consciousness or a highly-developed nervous system— and our collective God bleeds and is hurt by sin.

Perhaps the sin lies not in eating the meat but in the presumption and disrespect with which a meat animal is bred, imprisoned, and tortured on the way to the abattoir, and the overall effect of meat-farming on the cosmos. Perhaps the virtue is not in declining the eating of flesh but in the spirit of respect and gratitude in which any food is eaten.

Friday, February 24, 1989

I want to know if the temperature dropped below zero last night as predicted but I don't want radio or TV to disturb the sound pattern the cats and I have worked out for mornings— the pouring of catfood, the running of water, the hiss of steam and expansion sounds of coffee brewing. Then the discreet tick and crunch of catfood politely eaten, silently sipped coffee, the clicks and rush of furnace and traffic well outside our morning world.

...It is 1959. The light is pale and cool as we rise silently from the five beds lining the wainscoted walls of this mansion bedroom. I am ravenous. We follow the systems through the bathrooms and passages, still wordless, knot our variously-colored hair prissily at our napes and don our habits.

...Downstairs I stop in front of a wood and glass cabinet to unfold a small crisp veil from its shelf. It flutters and pulls at its bobby-pin mooring as I take my place in the tiny dark chapel, then settles silently with me. The red sanctuary candle burns perpetually and unswervingly in this unventilated room. Silence is broken by morning prayers spoken, and I am ravenous.

…We assemble before the stable-cum-garage and then step off, two by two, to attend mass at the cathedral, our parish church. My blood sugar drops but my jitters are not obvious as I walk. Inside I cannot kneel up straight, I prop myself against the pews before and behind.

…Seated in a carved high-backed throne of a chair before a long banquet table, I compose myself. While I'm still I'm fine but as a dish of hot boiled eggs is passed to me, my tremor reasserts itself. I clatter an egg into the bowl before me. Across the table and over the shoulders of sisters tapping on eggshells, a wall of open French doors frames a walled rose terrace beyond. A bouquet of roses, toast, coffee, incense, candlesmoke lingers in the morning light in which we are imbedded…

I leave the convent. Again.

…It is 1973. Now the old country farm-wife, I plunge robust and willing into all the grape vats I see. The house is shadowy and cool and smooth as glass until the children wake.

…We put away the traces of night and are off on a great adventure of creating, growing, conserving, learning. We are juicy and heavy with enthusiasm. Cut us and we will spurt quilts made, stories told, trees moved, sand castles built, water wells drilled, oceans of yogurt cultured, acres landscaped, bread birthed, fruits and vegetables preserved, concrete poured, paint applied. My feet are stained, my nails broken, my muscles large…

…It is 1965. Sunday afternoon. From my eighth floor room I look down on the patched and rotted roofs of flop-houses and boarded-up buildings, tottering offices, once respectable and dignified, now garish and pandering to any seeker of cheap rent or back-alley liaison. Gritty gray light seems nowhere to originate. A man slumps in a doorway—

that is, perhaps he is a man, perhaps he is slumped, perhaps that is a doorway…

Saturday, March 11, 1989

On Thursday evening I met a woman whose long-standing and active RA has been kept under control with a series of drugs I've never even heard of. She says her doctor is very well-informed and is always willing to try new things when she is willing. She has no deformity at all. Unfortunately when I called her doctor's office yesterday I learned that he's not accepting new patients right now—but I *am* on a waiting list so I'm filled with hope; maybe I've *finally* found the genius, M.D. I've been praying for!

I pull myself back to reality and then what I want is to stay curled around this pad on my knees, searching intently for something I expect to find there. As if I've narrowed my search to these few inches between my eye and my fingers, as if I expect truth to be a spider vein that I can follow on my pen to the mother lode.

Holy Saturday, March 25, 1989

My darling nephew, Carl John Nies, died last night at 9:05 p.m. He was almost eleven. He died of cancer.

> *It's spring. The door is open. I smell the fire. Full circle.*
> *I seek and I find*
> *an infinity of circles*
> *ending*
> *in an infinity of mirrors*
> *glinting back into my soul.*

If a phoenix is to rise from her ashes
her dehydrated loose bones
her atrophied tissues and scattered feathers
she must do so alone
from her soul outward
so that when she hits the air
her bones will have grown long and resilient
her soft parts unified, moist, vigorous, elastic
her feathers lush and shining
her wings and feet
strong and fleet.

A wounded phoenix is rightly abandoned
by those who would have her saved
who would themselves be wounded
in a rescue attempt: if she is to live
she must heal herself.

She must fan her spark
into breath
energy begun again.
She has nothing to lose
but a spark and no means
to extinguish it.

Sunday, March 26, 1989 — Easter

If there is no god
it must be that I am god
and I am not god.

I am a hostage to the rise and fall of RA and I can't seem
to escape it or even to placate it. The damage has become so

great again that my doctor is urging surgery on both hands and both feet within six months. I was hoping that things would improve somehow but my feet are so deformed now that I can barely walk. I've been wearing the most hideous orthopedic shoes which the kids and I call my "prunes"—and even *they* are no longer adequate to cushion my feet.

The ulnar deviation in both hands is causing immense pain and limitation. In addition to that, the extensor tendons of the outer two fingers on my right hand have been damaged or broken and I can no longer straighten those fingers so I must have tendon transplants. Will I have to have another round of surgery every four or five years???

I want to think about other things and plan for other things but always RA claims the best of my attention and energy. I want to change my line of work if I can, but I don't have the time or energy to even research the possibilities, so I suppose I wouldn't have the extra oomph that would be necessary to launch myself into another career. Maybe I should just forget about changing my work—but I strongly suspect it is partly the work I do, as well as my generalized fear, that keeps this disease so active.

> The path we take is so often spiral in shape. We cycle through patterns that bring us repeatedly back in the vicinity of whatever our nemesis is that we must meet and master....The heroine's journey is an individuation quest. Travelling this path, the heroine may find, lose, and rediscover what has meaning to her, until she holds onto these values in all kinds of circumstances that test her. She may repeatedly encounter whatever threatens to overcome her until finally the danger of losing her selfhood is over.
>
> – from *Goddesses In Every Woman,* by Jean Shinoda Bolen.

I must follow my own light even though I see that their lights illuminate their paths and even overflow onto mine. Still I must follow my light, my star.

> *God*
> *give me a seed crystal*
> *to grow my life on*
> *let your design reveal itself—my desperation*
> *tells me the design*
> *I've been living is not yours. I will*
> *look for it like*
> *easter eggs.*

Friday, April 28, 1989

Robert Assagioli writes that people experience their individuality in terms of *will,* rather than health or appearance or any other factor, which means that existence is identical with the capacity to express will.

If this is true—and it *does* seem true to me—then even though my life is dominated by RA, my frustration and dissatisfaction derives more directly from not doing what I want to do, what I'm called to do and, only insofar as RA limits me in that way, is it the seat of my discontent. The strongest limiting factor in my life is really my *fear* of committing myself to doing what I say I want to do— write—and taking the time and the steps to do that.

Should I commit myself to writing and look at my lack of time, my low energy, my need for a day job to pay the bills as mere *conditions* of my writing rather than as true barriers to it?

Wednesday, August 30, 1989

> *God is always*
> *just behind you can see her*
> *shadow, smell her*
> *breath, alas*
> *like two sides*
> *of a coin forever*
> *back to back*
> *you can't turn quickly enough*
> *to look her in the eye.*

Another year has begun. Rain goes back to school today; Kevin went back a week ago. He's taken up rock climbing; I don't want to think about that any more than I want to think about Rain jumping high hurdles.

Rain has completed her Girl Scout gold project, cleaning up a quarter-mile stretch of one of the many tributaries of the Rouge River. It has taken all spring and all summer and I couldn't begin to count the people who participated. I wonder if the river feels better without all those rotted tires, petrified shoes, blackened lumber, corroded beer cans, Skoal tins, fallen branches, molding potato chip bags, sodden tennis balls, slimy leather dog bones.

Last Friday I left my job at the machine tool company to take a job as comptroller at St. Victor's. I start Monday. I think I'll like the academic setting better than the boisterous world of machine tooling. And, who knows, maybe I'll take another look at the church.

Wednesday, November 1, 1989

One of the fringe benefits of working on a Catholic campus is the observance of holy days of obligation by closing classrooms and offices. Today is the feast of All Saints so, instead of driving into the blinding morning sun, I'm looking through my quiet window into a shadowy north, sliced right by those brilliant morning rays, at leafless trees festooned with last night's Halloween toilet paper.

The furnace blows sturdily and, for minutes at a time, I am warm and comfortable in my sprawl and sweats. Then pressure and discomfort begin to make themselves known, again, to my nervous system so I shift position slightly and therein lies the pain. Sometimes I prolong the interval of stillness but then the pain is that much greater and long-lived.

Saturday, November 4, 1989

I had my wrists injected with cortisone yesterday so I'm feeling much less pain. I did feel a few breath lapses and hints of palpitation—and fear of death as I was falling asleep last night. My stomach has been jittery but I've been hungry and energetic.

Sunday, November 12, 1989

The effects of the cortisone seem largely gone after only one week. Already yesterday my shoulders were again painful and their range of motion had decreased. My knees are feeling disjointed again. My hands and wrists are more painful and loose, *worse* than before the injection.

Sunday, November 19, 1989

Sunday morning quiet with a fresh layer of snow softening the sounds and brightening the whiteness. The furnace blows steadily then dozes. Brother Tom The Thanksgiving Turkey, thaws thoughtlessly in the garage, and calls to the cats who plead at the door.

I want to remember how cortisone affected me so I won't agree to it again. I feel generally jittery for days—especially my stomach. I'm even hungrier than usual. My face frequently becomes hot and red. I want to sleep a lot. I have many vivid, interesting, and memorable dreams—the only good effect other than the relief from pain, stiffness, and limitation.

I also want to remember that prescribed steroids are very dangerous in that frequent use can destroy my body's ability to produce natural steroids, and can actually damage my adrenals. Awaiting sleep, I become fearful of dying as I feel vague physical distress in my chest. I experience heartbeat irregularity several times daily, especially when I lie on my left side.

The last time I had injections in both wrists, they got immediately worse while everything else got immediately better. After two or three days my hands and wrists also improved but, by the end of the week, everything was worse than before the injections. Like gold salts and surgery, steroids are no panacea.

§

Thursday, March 8, 1990 — 6:49 a.m.

I'm having the first of this round of surgeries tomorrow morning so, for eight or nine months I'll have both the time and the circumstance to back up and regroup, to redesign my life. I can't just keep drifting and wishing as I have been for so long. I must make a clean, sharp turn and not worry about those shouting after me.

I left my work at the college less than fourteen hours ago and I never want to think about it again. These past months have been a trial return to the Catholic world I reluctantly left so many years ago, to see if I wanted to rejoin that stream of life, to see if it would now be compatible with what looks like truth to me. It didn't take long to realize that I can't, even as an employee, rejoin that stream—which I find to be more a backwater of less-evolved teachings about God, nature, power, women. I don't want to go back to my job on the twenty-third.

This time tomorrow I'll be lying braceletted, charted, tranquilized, and calm, swathed in green linen, on a pre-op gurney at University of Michigan Hospital.

Tuesday, March 13, 1990

When I clumped into the house yesterday and looked at the accumulation of mail, I was happy to see an envelope with the chancellor's return address and shocked when I opened the letter and a severance check fluttered to the floor! To be discharged while on authorized medical leave by a Catholic institution was something I would never have thought possible of Christian charity.

I see more clearly than ever now that outgrown beliefs must be finally if not tenderly laid to rest. There is no point in regretting that I haven't always had the knowledge I have today but outgrown companions and relationships, ideas and sentiments, must be retired when it's time. Past and present must be peacefully reconciled with each other and with truth.

Wednesday, March 14, 1990

It's 71° outside, I hear on the mid-day news. Because I've just had surgery on my feet my knowledge of outdoor conditions comes filtered through the TV or window glass but it's very hard to have a strong sense of a balmy spring day without opening a door to it, setting a foot in it.

I guess I could go out into the day, wearing my huge orthotic shoes over my great white bandages, and sit on the porch. Paranoid, I would feel threatened if I so allowed my vulnerability to show. But I can't experience spring locked up in the house and I can't get beyond paranoia and fear if I never challenge them.

Saturday, March 17, 1990

I've concluded, thousands of times, that I should unbuckle the harness and step out of the traces that bind me to those millstones conformity, custom, expectation, and fear; yet what mixed feelings I've had about my dismissal two days ago from a job I didn't want and was planning to leave.

I've felt cheated of due process, of being confronted by an accuser, of hearing specific charges and being allowed to answer those charges, of a clear advance warning. I've felt embarrassed, humiliated, that I've been publicly exposed to and at the mercy of a hostile, self-serving and hypocritical community. I've wanted to defend myself, to set the record straight, to punish for having had control snatched from my hands.

On the other hand, with the stroke of someone else's pen, I've been relieved of a job I didn't want and was planning to leave. And I've also been relieved of the odious obligation to orient my successor.

Why is it that I never see into the eye of the sun yet
learn everything solar
by reading the moon and hearing the tales of the stars?
Physicists know the body of God, but I guess at
Her form, only in myth.

Saturday, April 28, 1990 — with my right hand!

My right hand couldn't write for thirty-five days while it was
splinted and bandaged after the surgery and today it writes
again!

Since each finger has two, one extensor tendon was
transplanted from each of my inner two fingers to each of my
outer two fingers, so now I can extend those fingers again.
My right thumb joint was fused because it had so badly
deteriorated that it was bending backward and using a pen
was becoming difficult; it's still pinned with two giant hat pins.
The bony overgrowth on my ulna was removed and the bones
in my wrist and hand repositioned so the nerve along the
outside of my arm is no longer being pinched. Aside from the
itch and sting of healing, my hand is much more comfortable.

Thursday, May 17, 1990

The pins were finally removed from my toes yesterday so now,
after eight weeks, I can wear shoes again! They're orthopedic
shoes but they're not quite as ugly as my old *prunes*—we call
my new ones *raisins*. My thumb pins are gone too so I no
longer look like the poster child for orthopedic surgery.

Even in the out-patient waiting room, where most people
are sporting casts or splints or bandages, I've been a curiosity
with orthotic shoes on both feet, my right hand and forearm
in a resting splint and a gnarled left hand. I must have looked
like the wreck of the Hesperus! I wish I could have spared all

those curious people, trying so hard not to stare, their guarded glances, but somehow it didn't seem quite appropriate to stand, clear my throat, and launch into an oration on the ravages of RA.

Saturday, May 19, 1990

Another milestone. Rain looks so lovely and grown-up this evening in her senior prom ivory brocade, and Jason looks so handsome in his black tux, but I think of them more easily as kindergartners, or playing flute and trumpet in the band, as members of the track team. In only a few months they'll be off to different colleges.

Sunday, June 13, 1990 — Rain's graduation

The sun rose in a blaze of glory so by two when the ceremonies began it was sweltering in Ford Auditorium. The outdated air-conditioning system strained valiantly but failed miserably; there wasn't a dry body in the house, particularly among the graduates, in their brown nylon caps and gowns, and the orchestra, in black tie. Rain's commencement exercises were predictable, yet moving and wonderful.

After all the pomp and circumstance—the march across the stage to receive diplomas, the speeches and awards, the switching of the tassels, the tossing of the caps—like brown birds, the graduates fluttered back up the aisle, amid the thundering ovation of family and friends, on the first leg of their flight from our world.

I had a steroid injection so I could tolerate the ride to the auditorium and the long sit there. I'm still feeling post-surgically shaky and fragile; I hope it didn't show.

Monday, June 18, 1990 — first left-hand surgery

Excess bone was removed from my radius to relieve the pinching of the nerve that was causing numbness. In addition, a flexor tendon was transplanted from my ring finger to my thumb to enable me to bend it again, which I haven't been able to do for some time.

Monday, June 25, 1990 — second left-hand surgery

This time bony excess was removed from my ulna and my hand and wrist bones were repositioned to improve function and reduce deformity. I'm glad the surgeries are finally over.

Wednesday, August 15, 1990

All the pins and sutures and bandages have been gone for awhile now but rehabilitating my hands is still quite time-consuming. For weeks it was necessary to massage the surgical sites many times daily in order to prevent adhesions. Now I must go through a range of exercises several times daily to strengthen my hands and to keep the tendons flexible.

At first I thought the surgeon was kidding when he told me that I would have to *teach* the transplanted tendon in my left thumb how to behave like a thumb rather than like the ring finger from whence it came. It became obvious pretty quickly, however, that he wasn't kidding, and I had to spend long hours exercising and using my thumb to train it to stay in proper thumb position.

Rain has been keeping the house going and taking excellent care of me during this ordeal but I won't need much assistance by the time the kids leave for school. My brothers will be available to help me after that, if necessary.

I'm feeling so much better than I was before I began this round of surgery. I should be in excellent condition to start the job-hunting routine again. Fortunately, since I was discharged while on authorized medical leave, I have been eligible for unemployment compensation for part of the time I have been off work. But the money is getting thin so I'm actually looking forward to returning to work and paying off the debts I've accumulated.

At the moment I'm pretty happy about my writing effort because I've written reams during these months. I haven't tried to market anything but I will be able to do that on a part-time basis when I'm again working at an eight-to-five accounting job.

In fact, I wouldn't mind working overtime for awhile, not only to pay off my debts but to ease the pain of the absence of both children since in a matter of weeks I will be living alone, the mother emerita of adult children embarked on lives of their own.

I'm very excited to see Kev and Rain fly, yet reluctant to let them go. But so much of life is two-sided like a coin, or many-faceted like a crystal or a stone, or an optical illusion; to see another side it is necessary to abandon the security of clinging to the certainty of the first side. Once the second side is finally glimpsed, it's a bit easier to choose either side whole-heartedly or to choose to try to straddle two worlds.

Part of me is looking forward now to a simpler life, even a life alone, a more focussed life. My tides are calmer now than when I was younger and inclined to rush in and out, here and away, at most hours of the clock. Oddly, I'm entrained more with the moon now, beyond my fertile years, and I now instinctively keep her matins, her lauds, her vespers.

I dream on this peak
in some measure of leisure
and deny the fear that drives me yet
stills my cells, my joints, my poise, my choice
frozen, I straddle this watershed.

To one sunlit side blaze rainbow eddies
clouds of sweet warm sand
soft fruit, a sea of
brethren like daffodils or bunny
ears blowing in the wind.
On the other side cool
mists veil a drop fast
and precipitous white-lit flowing
fresh to the horizons of the stars.

I can yet stop and crawl out
onto an unpeopled space and nest
there among such others
as are washed nearby.

Saturday, September 22, 1990

Three days ago Rain was bereft of all comfort of remembering
why she chose a college in California, so far from home. She
was without hope that she might ever again be happy. She
realized that she had made a fatal choice, and could never
change her mind and come back home. She hung suspended
in mid-air as the flames of hell licked at her feet and angel
wings fluttered forever out of her reach.

Today she is giddy in the afterglow of welcoming speeches
and intimations of glories to come. Sleep deprivation and
physical hunger have been mislaid among the camaraderie of

new faces, myriad activities, and emancipation from parental presence.

She telephoned at six this morning to say that she's on her way to marching band practice (she'd planned not to join). By Thursday, when classes begin, she will have slept, eaten, spotted a clay foot or two—possibly at the end of her leg— and perhaps noticed that all living is choice.

Welcome to the class of '94.

Autumn officially begins today and this morning's sky already has the sharp edges of fall. Freshness prevails, as if all humidity and pollens and contaminants have fallen to an earth that will resorb them, along with man's other tailings too heavy to have become airborne. The earth breathes cool and calm, yet live and promising, catching her breath, preparing for rest under snows to come.

In the absence of a fireplace, I've taken to lighting a mass of candles morning and evening on the coffee table. Fire comforts me; it composes me and wards off evil spirits. It warms me. It reminds me of my power for good and for evil. My fire orients me to the earth from which I must draw my measure. My real context is not my house, my family, my company, my ego; my real context is the cosmos, my most extended self.

As I linger over cooling quenched candles and peer through the open window, between fluttering curtains, my thoughts wander undisciplined among chiseled white clouds on an Easter-egg blue sky. Ahhh—the comforts of coffee, sunshine, crisp breezes, soft clothing and simply abiding in a moment without agenda…

Monday, September 24, 1990

My body hurts. My job search is not going well. I miss Kev
and Rain. The news is as disturbing as ever.

The scabs have all been rubbed off my confidence again
and plasma beads up on the raw spots. I sip tea and my faux
fire crackles and glows hot upon my squatting knees.

Tuesday, September 25, 1990

Shy, Morning lingers in the shelter of the shadows spread out
to dry as traffic rushes and rumbles and jostles the day awake.
She calms me after another night of wrestling with my old
devils. Sometimes my psyche just can't relax with the fuzzy
new gods I'm considering—this heresy of abandoning a
perfectly serviceable occupation, accounting, for pie in the
sky, writing. Sometimes I wish someone would nail one of my
feet to the floor to establish for me a comfortable range and
predictable discomfort—yet isn't that what I rail most against?

What do I really want? I want to offer something that is
uniquely mine to give to a world that is, like me, hungry and
searching. I want to offer food, or words, or both, for what
they're worth—definitely not as last words, last supper, but
only as feet under creations' endless table. I don't want to be
a guru or a savior—just a cousin sharing an hour or a meal.

I want to slip the surly bonds of the patriarchy which
requires the two-thousand-hour work year with no hope of
sabbatical until enforced retirement. I wish for the demise
of the system which, to those who are temporarily AWOL,
promises penalties upon return to orthodoxy and punishment
when comes that enforced retirement.

I want to not feel the hot breath, the fevered surveillance
of other captives who haven't tried to escape and whose
anxiety grows each day I'm away. Nearly everyone in my
world believes that the only possible agenda for my time is to

consume it in earning as much as humanly possible and tending my stuff. Even I sometimes believe this way down deep in the jittery cells of my stomach, the tense tissues of my lungs and throat, who haven't been permanently convinced that my time is *my* time, my body is *my* body, my life is *my* life.

I continually look for new truth, total truth without paradox, and what I find is changing perspectives, oxymoronic echoes now from my pen, now from your mouth, now from the heart and soul and entrails of all to infinity.

My journal and my health are books of my shadows, reality as projected onto the walls of my personal sky. They are grim gargoyles and looming grotesques, as well as totems and gulfs of blooming light.

New expressions of ancient truths sometimes *do* flow from my pen, but rarely after being awakened from sound sleep or struck dumb from my horse by a lightning bolt. Mostly my paraphrases or restatements or syntheses are lying around loose in my mind when I drift awake into morning or they are delayed reactions to the teachings of others which I've integrated into the body of my reality. All of us are unwitting plagiarists, that is, arcs of the eternal circle of truth, I think, or shards of the shattered hologram of God.

Wednesday, November 7, 1990

The first few snowflakes of the season huddle on the window sill but they'll be on their way back to the sea within the warming hour. A soft warm presence passed by as Lickie deliberated on the doorsill about the relative merits of inside and outside. Ultimately, she chose the doorsill and I seem to be stuck there.

Monday, November 12, 1990

Yesterday morning November smoothed off the last of the gold crumbs of Indian Summer and folded fall quietly away. In turn, she shook blustery winds, and ten minutes of snowflakes swirling madly into my windshield, from the previews of December and hard winter waiting their turns.

This morning all is in retreat, resting until the onset of holiday celebration and talk of celebration, cooking and eating and talk of cooking and eating, gifts and talk of gifts, love and talk of love and then, reforming, renewing, rebirth in the slow, low winter sun surely incubating another spring beneath the snow.

My tiny fire weaves and stretches companionably in the faint morning stir, a light witness to my arrival at this new sunrise. A pinkish halo tucked behind the trees and houses on the horizon rises slowly as if somewhere it's being infused with hot air and soon we'll all be riding on the wind suspended by this rosy donut. Suddenly a curtain drops and all is November again; serious snowfall should begin anytime now—yet water puddles on the black-top outdoors.

...now I snug up my makeshift shawl as a cold wind whines through the vents and leaks in my tent. The cloudy sky is so close I might touch the heavy black cloud hovering like a monstrous mushroom cap over huddled houses and shivering trees on a Thanksgiving late afternoon as I shake crumbs from an overstuffed tablecloth spotted with wine and cranberry, symbols of another season wrested from Nature and jarred and potted in the cellar. Only rarely does She rain manna or fruit drops or deliverance—mostly She offers prizes to be won in a friendly tug-of-war. Under this same black umbrella, the sharp wind freshens me as I step from the humid kitchen, sluggish in its heart...

Burning soft and quiet, my little fire soothes me with its invisible smoke. Shy morning light rearranges the shadows around me and overrides the silence.

I paid off the last $149.75 to University of Michigan Hospital. Now I own my refurbished joints free and clear.

Tuesday, February 19, 1991

For oil, in the civilized and enlightened year of 1991, the United Nations are killing people by the thousands. The air war rages on but the ground war hasn't started yet because the UN forces wish to take advantage of two of Nature's most reliable characteristics—high tide and new moon— to maximize military advantage, the commentator, a retired general, confides to all the TV world. I can't believe this war is happening even though I spend every available moment watching it on television.

Since warfare is one of the most primitive and oldest of vices, it doesn't seem any more outdated to note that this month is dedicated to one of the oldest of goddesses, Sophia, the Greek goddess of peace, rebirth, and wisdom. According to another tradition, the sun entering Pisces tomorrow calls for a celebration of intuition and harmony. What irony it would be if person-to-person combat would begin on the twenty-second, the ancient Roman feast of Concordia, a time when no one was allowed to carry a feud any further into the year.

Saturday, March 9, 1991

On my deathbed I'll regret it if I have never made a concerted effort to write professionally, even though I've written for pleasure since childhood. Writing thousands of journal pages has often been therapeutic as well as helpful in organizing my thoughts and plans. Once again, I vow to submit some of my writing as soon as I'm feeling better.

My RA has been flaring terribly for weeks and I'm weak as a kitten; walking even a few yards is exhausting. Fortunately, since late December I've been self-employed and doing the work of my two accounting clients at home, so I can control most of my life and no one else knows the extent of my physical difficulty unless I tell them.

Tuesday, March 12, 1991

My arms are incredibly painful. Perhaps that's because they're unsupported and my morning aspirin hasn't kicked in. I've always consoled myself with the fact that I've never lost my ability to use a pen or a keyboard, however else I may have been physically limited or disabled. But I see now that despite my many and varied efforts at cure, my fingers and toes continue to grow fixed at ever sharper angles. Just now I have pain at the base of my left thumb and slight dislocation in my left shoulder and holding a pen is excruciating. Typing might be more comfortable than using a pen.

I'm recently aware of a new and surprising *aversion* to writing. Yet I don't want to die with my only claim to fame being the fact that I raised two thinking children. I want to leave something concrete that is only mine.

Wednesday, April 24, 1991

I was finally able to get in to see my friend's doctor. He did a thorough examination and was appalled at the damage to my joints, particularly my ankles and my shoulders. Let's see: I have rheumatoid arthritis, osteoarthritis (now called degenerative joint disease) and probably a history of gout, fibrositis, and myositis—what, no heart disease? He prescribed methotrexate, a drug that is used primarily in the treatment of leukemia patients. He also suggested I stop using aspirin and use Naprosyn instead. Here's hoping…

Kevin is training for a Memorial Day bike marathon and spends some weekends mapping caves in southeastern Wisconsin while Rain runs the foothills and plays frisbee golf and roller-blades around Palo Alto; my only sport is bare-faced, flat-out, shameless *athlete envy*.

Wednesday, May 22, 1991

The new drugs are working; physically I'm feeling a lot better already but I almost don't care because today Kevin found out that he too has RA. He's not as upset as I am, it seems; I am heartbroken.

He'd been having problems with his knees but we attributed it to the strenuousness of his weekend biking and rock-climbing and caving. However, even after he stopped doing those things the pain and inflammation and redness didn't go away so when the semester ended he consulted my rheumatologist who made the diagnosis.

RA is three times more common in women than in men so I'm a little surprised that Kev has come up with it. I wonder whether it's a contagious disease which he got from me or a genetic trait inherited from me or possibly from my mom, since lupus is very like RA.

Tuesday, June 30, 1991

Day five after a ten-hour storm that knocked out the electrical power supply to one quarter of the state...

How fiercely a Michigan summer storm shreds the black northern sky, slaps sheets of water hard against buildings, her high winds menacing even the sturdiest trees braced against the assault. Small things—plants, toys, lawn chairs, debris— are winnowed in wave after wave of rising and falling winds. Then stillness. Then silence. Then without warning another blast of huge cold drops hammers the torn earth, the black sky lit brilliant yet again, thunder splits the air, lightning slashes an endless afternoon.

How sweet it is to walk after midnight in the storm's tranquil wake and see everything nearly as clearly as day. How bright is the night without the street lights and commercial lights and house lights extinguished by the storm. How insignificant is candlelight and lantern light amid the greatness of starlight in a sky now cleared of cloud and thunder.

How serene are the post-storm day sounds: the hiss and hum, buzz and thrum, murmur and peep of insects usually drowned out by the roar of the lawn care equipment of greater suburbia; of hand-washed laundry flapping gently on makeshift clothes lines when all the washers and dryers of the neighborhood lie helpless without their electrical or gaseous motivation; the small sounds of minor household chores being done with hand tools while power tools are similarly crippled. How soft is the sound of conversation among folks, convinced finally of the futility of blustering at the power company customer relations representative and resigned at last to simply waiting, then listening less and less to the battery-powered radio for news of the ETA of the utility workers. How reluctantly-made are the forays in the car to the store miles down the road where all is normal, where electricity flows like water and supplies are sold.

How delicious are the makeshift meals cooked with little fuel and served with plain ceremony and eaten with slow appreciation and enjoyment. How deep is the harsh pleasure of washing dishes and bodies in cold water in the heart of the city, in quiet natural light, without the sound of anything mechanical.

How comforting it is to hear the night sounds: the breathing of breezes through bushes and trees, the voices of night birds and night insects, the chirp of crickets and songs of frogs, the mysterious swishes and thumps, newly audible in the absence of TVs and radios and stereos and VCRs, dishwashers and refrigerators, air conditioners and fans, the dull roar of routine and complexity.

How full of pure joy is being in the bright night outdoors, barefoot in the dewy grass, until time to go to bed by feel or candlelight and then to share the open-window small sounds of neighbors bedding down in dark houses; to hear the quiet of the country or campground in the middle of a closely-populated neighborhood with all the comforts of home in the city—except electricity.

Wednesday, July 10, 1991

The effectiveness of the methotrexate has diminished, but my doctor said that's not unusual and he increased the dosage.

Thursday, July 18, 1991

I'm heartsick again. After weeks of back, wrist, and leg pains, Rain's doctor in California gave her a diagnosis of ankylosing spondylitis, another auto-immune disease, and today she got a second opinion from my rheumatologist who confirmed the original diagnosis. Have I passed this god-awful tendency on to my children? I feel so guilty and, worse, I can't stand the idea of them having to live their entire adult lives as I have lived mine for the past twenty years.

Sunday, August 25, 1991

Like convent Sundays. A few cars pass. A car alarm sounds briefly. Shadows of the hedge are long and wet. Birds chatter over breakfast. Neighbors' cars pose red, cream, navy on the parking area. Another car passes by. The warm cat lays limply on her left side along my leg and sleeps the sleep of the fed, the loved, the secure. My beloved son speeds toward college with his dad—they may be negotiating Chicago about now. My beautiful daughter sleeps California dreams, 5:30 in her world, a butterfly waiting for her wings to dry.

Friday, August 30, 1991

I've had to have another increase in my methotrexate dosage and now I'm combining it with gold salts injections. My doctor assures me this has been tested enough to not be especially dangerous even though it isn't often done. I hope he's right.

Friday, November 29, 1991

My cortege threads
inconsolable
among upside-down picnic tables, spindly, helpless
isolated
from domino lines of randy others
mounting one after another.

Green lakes, desolate, glacial
mourn hills vacant
of Taps blown.
Birch trees quake a secret tremolo
praying desperate vespers
hover over
shedding corpses shutting down.

Spiny saplings, nubile, mobile, whip
in precision drill
under the baton of mad snow devils.

My procession cants wearily upward to
dormancy.

A piper patrols the barren crest
and rips the heat from my gutted chest
wheezing sadness, pain
then blows into my frozen hands
until I smell pine and tangerine.

Monday, December 2, 1991

The methotrexate/gold combination is barely working any more and I'm getting nervous about the results of my liver studies, although my doctor reassures me that elevated values are to be expected and are nothing to worry about.

Friday, December 20, 1991

Rain arrived home from college for Christmas break. It's so good to have her here. I wish Kev were here too but his last final is not until the twenty-third.

Rain has invited me to go back to Stanford with her on the sixth to see her school and I think I'll go. This combination of methotrexate and gold salts has almost ceased to work and there is nothing else for me, according to my doctor. I'm going to ask him to give me a steroid injection so I can make this trip in comfort since it will probably be my only chance to see Rain's college.

Just in time, feathery snow has blanketed everything while Rain and I were busy with dinner and getting her settled and catching up. She's feeling good and her back and her joints bother her only occasionally; she takes buffered aspirin on those occasions.

The cortisone that was pumped into my knees yesterday has spread through my body, thirsty as a sponge, delivering blessed relief from pain and limitation. Since I can expect the cortisone to hold up reasonably well for at least two weeks, I'm even planning to visit other friends in Oregon when I travel west on the sixth. I'll go out in a blaze of travelling glory, so to speak, since my treatment prospects, once the gold/methotrexate combination finally fails, are *zero*. The only alternative then will be steroids—and I'm not going to take that route more than very occasionally. But, like Scarlett O'Hara, I'll think about that tomorrow, or when the time comes. Right now, I'm on hiatus from ill health and I'm on my way to California and points west! *Yee-hah!*

⚘

A Chain of Summer Lightning

Hope, Alternative Medicine, and Success

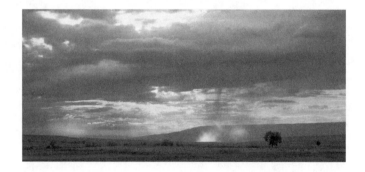

A Chain of
Summer Lightning

Tuesday, January 21, 1992

I'M IN LOVE AGAIN! I've been to the San Francisco Bay area
and I am hers. Her lush vegetation, soft golden hills and deep
green mountains, the wide Pacific probing with marshy fingers
deeply inland, her perfume of eucalyptus and coffee, and her
happy informality have all called my name.

I've decided to move to the Bay area but I have another
health crisis to address first. The effects of the cortisone have
worn off, the gold and methotrexate combination is not
working any more, even at the higher dosage, and now I'm
frightened because the results of my liver studies are almost
off the scale. I'm afraid to again increase the dosage as Dr. W.
has recommended. Now is definitely the time to think about
other alternatives.

One of the most serendipitous parts of my trip was
meeting Sonia, who'd had RA and who'd been on saturation
aspirin therapy, as I had been, and who was healed—or cured,
or relieved, or whatever the correct term would be—of RA
as an unexpected result of a political fast she'd undertaken.
She said she simply woke up on the morning of the sixth or

seventh day of her water-only fast (no aspirin) and the disease was gone! And it has not returned in over ten years.

Sonia referred me to her friend, Jean, in New Mexico, who is an herbalist and nutritionist. We had a lengthy telephone consultation in which she gave me a list of dietary changes to make after I undertake a fast of at least six days. She told me to eliminate all meat, milk, sugar, white flour, coffee, black tea, nightshades (potatoes, tomatoes, peppers, eggplant, tobacco) and commercially processed foods. She suggested that I see what's available at the public library and local book stores and to read everything I can find on the subjects of fasting, vegetarianism, and alternative medicine in general, so today I begin studying.

I'm aware that I'm considering heresy here since the Arthritis Foundation's published "quack remedies" list includes special diets (do-eat, don't-eat, no-nightshades, oriental, allergy, elimination), as well as herbal treatments, home remedies, folk remedies, metabolic therapy, homeopathy, acupuncture, shiatsu, and "bizarre methods" (injecting salts of heavy metal is not bizarre?).

…I dream up a California goddess to bless my effort… she's barefoot, in baggy knickers and rolled-up sleeves, with long gray hair French-braided down her back. She pushes a battered baby grand into position on a bare wood floor in a room hung with drying flowers…the walls are lined with tables laden with steaming food and melting ices, and laughing people fling their shoes under the tables as violin and guitar strings are tuned in a corner…my goddess lounges, cabaret singer style, atop the piano and pronounces a blessing: *"Laissez les bon temps rouler!"* Let the good times roll!

My reading informs me that vegetarianism has been around at least since the sixth century when Pythagoras mentioned it in his work. It even has an institutional history; in 1847 a Vegetarian Society was formed in England and in 1889 the Vegetable Federal Union was founded here. There was once even a political party of vegetarians, I read in *Fasting: The Phenomenon of Self-Denial* by Eric N. Rogers. According to Rogers, a list of famous vegetarians would include Jean Jacques Rousseau, Leo Tolstoy, George Bernard Shaw, Annie Besant, and Mohandas Gandhi, so I'm already in pretty good company.

Significantly, the last of my solstice candles, lit one month ago today, burns low as I make three solemn vows to myself: I'm going to move, I'm going to be well, I'm going to write. A mere puddle now, my candle burns no less, gives no less light at this moment than on Winter Solstice a month ago when she was first lit. I'm glad for her company and her symbolism.

Monday, February 3, 1992 — 7 a.m.

An oversized furry black slug, in the person of the Burmese she-cat, Licorice, wheezes beside me as I sip the first of numbered cups of coffee. Outside these warm walls, pairs of headlights push through the cold Michigan dark. Within my skin, all is pain.

The entire back of my body ached enough to prevent sleep, so I left my bed before I was refreshed—as usual. Sitting is better. But then my hips and thighs ache. Standing is better. Except that the weight of my unsupported arms begins to dislocate the bones in my shoulder joints. The spurs on the soles of my feet impinge upon nearby nerve endings and my feet shriek for the relief of walking. Walking is better. Except that my hips begin to gripe and my knees quickly become weary and strained and unstable. Shifting position every few minutes is best.

My wrists ache with writing—or resting. My neck strains as I bend over my pad. I have a headache which never goes away but merely moves from spot to spot—this morning it's just below my crown. The throb in my left ankle is punctuated occasionally by sharp stabs; it's been hot, red, and fluid-engorged for about ten days now. My calves and knees ache.

I rise to pour cup #2 and a sore and tender muscle seems to detach from my kneecap and peel up my thigh. My knees creak. Back again on the sofa, my left palm tugs discordantly as its components—muscles, tendons, ligaments, bones—designed to work in concert, instead oppose each other. My hand feels as if it's breaking apart. And it looks so, too, as my hand bones deviate about 20° toward my thumb while my fingers deviate about 45°in the other direction. Some days I can almost see my hand in the act of drifting away from the normal straight line of my ulna.

Still, today is a good day. I feel energetic. I'm not depressed. No joint is totally dislocated. Although my entire body aches, joints and soft tissue alike, only my left ankle is relentlessly painful. My digestive system is completely comfortable, my breathing is comfortable, I can hear, and I can write.

> *Cramped limbs, cocooned in limitation*
> *damp and mildewed brain, balled up in despair*
> *open, unfold, expand*
> *like compressed sponges thrown back to the sea;*
> *a dehydrated self blooms*
> *into the sun.*

My furry familiar sleeps under the stereo as the colorless morning proceeds toward nine and I pour cup #4 and ponder this treason I'm considering. My back aches.

When other animals are sick or wounded, they often don't eat and they drink only a little water. Neither do they go to work as usual. Instead, they curl up in a cave or a corner, a cool spot or a sunbeam, until they feel better or they die. We humans, on the other hand, punch in as usual after having chemically jump-started, super-charged, and dynamited our ailing bodies, or anesthetizing to the point of premature embalming; we live fast, we die young, we leave beautiful corpses. Body and/or soul don't want to move? Not to worry—take a pill—let's rock!

My ragged copy of Adele Davis' *Let's Get Well* reads that fasting and severe calorie restriction "are each such severe stress that the adrenals are left exhausted, a characteristic of which is continuous low blood sugar and its accompanying ravenous appetite and craving for sweets…If animals are deprived of food, or fasted, and hence no protein is given, the stress is so severe that ulcers develop within three days…during the severe stress of several weeks of fasting, the amount of uric acid in the blood of obese patients became increasingly higher until some developed gout."

Well, I can ignore the fright that last quote induced in me because I'm not thinking of fasting for several weeks and I'm not obese. I note that *Let's Get Well* was written in 1965 so I'm wondering about the currency of the research cited—but I'm not going to *dismiss* the warning.

In *The Nature Doctor,* H.C.A. Vogel writes, "One of the best remedies to maintain general well-being is fasting… When a person fasts the body has an opportunity to rid itself of accumulated harmful metabolic wastes." So—another war of the experts. As usual, when the authorities seem equally credible, I can pick the one whose findings most suit my own prejudices and hope for the best.

In *Natural Health, Natural Medicine* Andrew Weil writes,

> Fasting owes its effectiveness to a basic fact of physiology. The digestive organs are the largest and bulkiest in the body, and their routine operations consume large amounts of energy. The simple act of not eating rests this system and frees up much of that energy for the body to use in healing. Fasting means taking in nothing other than water (or water and herbal teas with no calories). Restricting yourself to liquids, fruit, or fruit juice is not fasting. These are special diets that have particular benefits but do not produce the same results as fasting.
>
> Short-term fasting alters both consciousness and physiology. It is a good home remedy for colds, flus, infections, and toxic conditions of all kinds…I have seen long-term fasting produce complete remissions of diseases that resisted all other treatments: bronchial asthma, rheumatoid arthritis, ulcerative colitis….Long-term fasting should be done only in a facility staffed by experienced health professionals.

Tuesday, February 4, 1992 — 6:15 a.m.

Pain hasn't awakened me but it prevents the sleep my head still struggles for. My ankle throbs; there is no comfortable position. On my back, the back side of my body feels raw; on my side, my shoulders feel crushed, my hips ache, my knees smart. My left calf feels tight and sore and swollen.

I sit up and all is stiff. My thumbs throb. My compromised wrist bones feel inadequate to support the weight of my hands. My head aches. The place where my neck joins the back of my head feels engorged and creaks loudly. Thank goodness for hot water which steams my filmy eyes open, my brain awake.

Her Royal Highness, Queen Licorice, having breakfasted at five, now summons me, the doorkeep, to let her out into a breezy faux spring morning—no basement litter box for her except when ice and snow promise frostbite or worse. The snow has all but disappeared except for a few patches that lie always shaded from the sun so much in evidence of late; the air temperature is enough above freezing for Lickie to venture beyond our world of humidified forced air and incandescent light. A few vehicles hustle through the crossroads outside my window.

Cantilevered off the edge of the sofa, I'm more comfortable. I sip cup #2 and push back. Oops, that makes my thighs ache. I lean forward to write and my shoulders and neck hurt. Ah, well, all living is choice, isn't it? Somehow the coffee consoles me. Coffee will be the most difficult sacrifice.

I'm not ready to give up anything more just yet but when I'm ready, my plan is to do a distilled-water-only fast and cleansing enema routine for awhile. Then I'll add diluted fresh juices, one at a time. Later, I'll break my fast with raw fruit, raw vegetables, raw seeds, raw nuts. Eventually, I'll add cooked grains and some oils, and move slowly toward a full diet according to Jean's recommendations.

Wednesday, February 5, 1992 — 5:51 a.m.

My ankle throbs. I try to soothe it by stroking and my fingers find something unfamiliar; a flat rectangular plate has formed on the bone. And another nodule, this one the size and shape of a half-grape, has formed on my Achilles tendon; I've had both such formations elsewhere on my body—elbows, right shin, soles, upper arms, fingers—but these two are new. The outsides of my legs ache insistently, my calf burns. Forget sleeping.

The coffee level in the can is going down; there's enough left for four or five days perhaps. As I pour I'm comforted by the aroma, the steam, the heated cup, by the morning ritual of brewing coffee and settling into writing position. I love the flavor of coffee. I love the stimulation of coffee, the drug that starts me breathing in the morning.

My wrists ache. My knees ache. My legs feel heavy, fatigued. I wonder if this is due to poor circulation yet I doubt it because my feet and toes are warm. The tendons in the front of my neck are sore and cold. All in all, not too bad a morning. I've had thousands much worse.

Although I'd largely given up on fresh milk many months ago, I didn't seriously begin to reduce the large amount of cheese and sour cream in my diet until just about three weeks ago after my consultation with Jean. My better mornings began about a week ago and since then I've reduced my daily aspirin intake from six to four to two to none at all for the last two days. And I've skipped two doses of methotrexate now. Although the level of pain has been about the same, it's obvious to me that there's been improvement since I changed my diet, especially since I've been taking less medication to kill the pain and reduce the inflammation. In addition, I've been eating more raw food. Still, my own devil's advocate, a week is not a long time; these improvements may be coincidental.

Madame L. flows from her sleeping comma position to an eagle spread to study me for a moment, then slips back into the exhausted morning sleep of the nightwalker. The world outside my window seems poised on a windless threshold among patches of shrunken snow and unmelted salt lumps strewn over the drive.

Ah! Sun arrives! And with her, other dimensions, shadows, hints, possibilities, warmth, promise. I am excited, exhilarated,

yet vaguely fearful. Of what? That I'm contemplating some
mortal sin, that I'll burn forever in hell if I die unforgiven by
some messiah, M.D. who couldn't cure my disease but who
nonetheless claimed my disease as only his to cure or not to
cure? Am I still illogically fearful that medical orthodoxy is
right and that investing a week or so in doing practically
nothing at all about my disease will, at last, be the thing that
seals my fate forever?

Is it rational to fear that, although my body has withstood
and even *responded* to years of massive doses of aspirin which
made me deaf to nearly everything but the constant ringing
in my ears, or the NSAIDs that gave me worse ulcers than
aspirin, or injections every two weeks of a salt of a heavy
metal, or injections of steroids, or a cancer chemotherapy
drug that made my hair fall out by the brushful and my liver
go crazy, or hours and hours of surgery—actual cutting and
pasting—not to mention the hours in recovery rooms and days
in hospital beds, it cannot withstand a week of no solid food
and no medication?

Thursday, February 6, 1992

My knees ache and crunch when I rise—"crepitus," my
physician calls the particles that move around in my joints but
I call them gravel. My knees have felt much better for months
now but, for the months before I started the methotrexate,
they were a source of genuine agony, swollen almost to the size
of softballs, hot to the touch, partially dislocated. Methotrexate
and gold salts injections have made my knees almost normal
for several months now; even today, they're still much better
than they were at their worst, yet recently they've been more
painful than they've been in months. I'm so disappointed that
the benefits have dwindled while the dangers have multiplied

and now this is no longer a prudent treatment; liver for joints is not a reasonable trade.

Suddenly my shoulders are more comfortable than they've been. For months, they've felt hunched, as if drawn up by shrinking tendons or ligaments, or by scar tissue. I would consciously try to relax them but it never helped more than a little and only for a few seconds. Today they're relaxed without effort, although my range of motion is still severely limited. I can't reach the cup shelf, for instance, four inches above eye level, and I can't scratch the itchy spot on the back of my neck without propping my elbow on the arm of the sofa.

Periods of bodily comfort and pleasure are only occasional with this disease, thus surprising and delicious when they do occur. In a way undreamed of back in the good old days before RA, I savor a good day, a warm shower, fresh clothing, soft socks, sitting comfortably, a good night's sleep, walking easily to the mailbox.

It's ironic that when I was a child my dad was often annoyed by my running when most people would walk, being hyperactive where many would relax, moving when he would sit still, reading while others were sleeping. "You drive everything into the ground," he would say, and he was right. I was very active physically as well as mentally until I was stricken with this disease.

Now I must choose my activities very carefully and I'm able to do only about a quarter of what I did before the onset of this disease, so limited has been my energy and so great my discomfort and the damage to my joints. Often, on the evenings when the kids were staying overnight with Bob, after my post-divorce return to salaried work when they were seven and five, I'd arrive home from work at about 6:30, eat some cold cereal while talking on the phone with Kev and Rain, and be asleep by 8:30 because I was so exhausted. Now my energy level is high but the pain and stiffness linger on. For over three years I've been unable to tolerate the eighty-mile airport round-trip when Kev and Rain were leaving for or returning from college.

Friday, February 7, 1992

Continents and archipelagos of stale snow float seas of black lawn as Licorice slides out into the unseasonably warm morning. I linger at the open door to greedily gulp the spring air. A very good morning to start a fast.

Pain wraps around my left calf and my ankles throb. My feet ache dully as I sit, sharply as I pad sock-footed around the kitchen, dispensing catfood and *not* making coffee. My legs sting and throb as if infected. My head seems entirely too heavy for my creaking, straining neck; I try to sit up straighter as I write but that doesn't help. My spine feels like it's compressing, telescoping into itself and into my pelvis. My hands and wrists ache. All the parts which come into contact with the sofa hurt. The base of my skull hurts. My whole back aches. My shoulders complain when I hunch to write—and when I straighten. My knees strain and crunch as I raise and lower myself. I'm drowsy but I can't sleep longer; the pressure from the mattress, even from my light comforter, keeps me awake. I'm hungry.

I don't know how hungry I am for food itself, but I know I'm hungry for my morning ritual, the warmth and flavor and stimulation of coffee. The promise of coffee has been for years my consolation prize for having to get out of bed unrefreshed and blurry-eyed; coffee has been my shot of adrenalin in a weary body, a jump-start out of exhaustion, an energy transfusion. I miss coffee already; I feel much as I felt on all those nothing-after-midnight mornings while I waited to be wheeled into surgery, deprived and anxious with some gnawing thing in the pit of my stomach. Thankful, I realize that I won't be awakening, many hours hence, in some recovery room, confined to casts, splints, and gauze. And I can drink water.

I'm going to drink distilled water for at least three days, I think now, but I want to intuitively control the timing. At various points I'll add vegetable broth and juices, then slowly break my fast with whole raw foods. I'm also going to do the enemas—*ugh*—twice daily—but I have strong reservations about that; other animals don't do enemas, even though they do fast when they're ailing. But then, other animals in the wild don't usually abuse their bodies with junk food and junk chemicals; although domestic animals will if their owners are unwise enough to provide them.

Even though Hippocrates said, "Let food be thy medicine," I'm quite excited about starting a fast because; the more I read the more hopeful I become. According to Herbert M. Shelton in *Fasting Can Save Your Life,* "Fundamentally and primarily the cause of arthritis is toxemia…symptoms are the result of toxic saturation…the primary irritation leading to the abnormal changes in the joints is due to the presence in the blood and lymph of unstable toxic material accumulating for months and years in one who is enervated. These sufferers are always heavy eaters." Aha!

In *Staying Healthy With Nutrition,* Elson M. Haas writes that most chronic and degenerative diseases result from *overnutrition* rather than malnutrition or under-nutrition; it's certainly obvious that most Americans are at least overfed, if not well-fed. This same author says that fasting is a preventive for many diseases such as athersclerosis, hypertension and heart disease, allergies, diabetes, and cancer. He writes that most Americans eat too much protein, too much fat, too much food of all kinds, and too often. Several other authors suggest that

eating itself is an allergy-addiction; could that be true? I
wonder if the two biggest industries, after food production
and distribution, are medicine and weight reduction. Haas
writes, "We all need to return to the cycle of a daily fast of
12-14 hours overnight until our morning 'break-fast,' and
then find our own natural pattern of food consumption.
This usually means one main meal and two lighter ones. For
low-weight, high-metabolism people, two larger or three
moderately sized meals are probably needed." He calls fasting
"nature's doctor and knifeless surgeon."

Shelton makes the observation that, "Every normal habit
indulged to satiety and every abnormal habit produces disease."
In recent years I've heard many similar statements made about
findings in nutrition and exercise research. In particular, I recall
reading in the news several times a few years back that the
ideal would be to always leave the table still just a little hungry,
that the healthiest and longest-living people are those who get
just barely enough to eat of wholesome 'peasant food.'

Certainly that is the moral guidance offered by many
religious counselors and often by lay counselors as well.
Apparently the old saw, "Too much of a good thing…"
is true in all realms of life.

According to Shelton, arthritis develops in predisposed
individuals and "represents an impaired state of nutrition in
addition to the common toxemia. The calcium deposits and
stone formation that are part of the disease indicate that the
nutritional perversion is similar to, if not identical with, that
which is back of the formation of gall stones, kidney stones,
hardening of the arteries, deposits of lime on the valves of the
heart, deposits in the feet in gout, and the formation of stones
in other parts of the body."

It seems that the body has such amazing recuperative and
regenerative powers that it is usually able to heal itself of even

gross abuses without medical intervention or, sometimes, in spite of medical intervention. When recovery is not occurring naturally, fasting gives the body an opportunity to relieve itself of toxic accumulations without the interference of routine digestion and continued ingestion of potentially toxic foods and medicines. Fasting can be the first step in starting over dietarily and then doing it properly.

I've wondered whether fasting might be more difficult for me than for other people since I seem to actually *need* all the food I consume; I eat like the proverbial field hand and I don't gain weight. I've wondered whether I might become thin as an anoretic, or permanently lose my appetite and in fact become anoretic. And other people with whom I've discussed my intention to fast are very concerned that I will have no protein intake.

I've wondered about both of those issues too but I've learned from my reading that anorexia is not primarily a physical health issue; it's primarily a psychological issue stemming from an abnormal need for control in a person who feels she has no control over anything in her life. I've also learned that the human need for protein is considerably lower than had been accepted for years and that our bodies, in Shelton's words, "contain sufficient nutriment to hold out, in most instances, for prolonged periods, especially if they are conserved and not wasted. In the blood and lymph, in the bones, and especially in the marrow of the bones, in the fat of the body, in the liver and other glands, and even in the individual cells that make up the body, are stores of protein, fat, sugar, minerals, and vitamins which may be drawn upon... Even thin individuals carry a reserve of food in their tissues, to tide them over periods of abstinence. These people too may safely fast for varying periods." He also wrote that arthritis "...sufferers are always heavy eaters."

All of the experts I've read agree that gastric irritation, which the faster perceives as hunger, ceases often on the second day of the fast or certainly by the fourth day. Well, that's good news.

The authorities I've read are very clear in their statements that it isn't the fasting itself that does the healing; it's the elimination of toxins by fasting that allows the body to heal itself when it hasn't been able to do so while eating as usual; however, one writes that, because almost every adult has such a great accumulation of toxic debris stored in fatty tissue, lengthy fasts are no longer safe without medical monitoring. Nonetheless, the list of chronic conditions that resolve themselves during and after a fast is impressive: eczema, varicose ulcers, asthma, colitis, amoebic dysentery, sinusitis, bronchitis, psoriasis, migraine, Reynaud's disease, kidney and bladder stones. Most of the authorities say fasting's effectiveness derives not from what it *does* but from what it *doesn't* do, that it merely provides an ailing body the opportunity to do for itself what it was designed to do.

Sunday, February 9, 1992 — 7:30 a.m. Day 3

Vegetable broth—*ugh!* I'm not going to finish it. By mid-evening yesterday, my energy and strength were both fairly high but I continued to sit, talk, and watch TV so I think the leg pains I've had since then are from lack of exercise rather than from anything more pathological.

11:30 a.m.

I can't believe it!!! I have almost no pain! After only a little over 48 hours fasting! I've had no gold injections for nearly three months now, no methotrexate for eleven days, no aspirin for about five days, and at this moment I have virtually no pain. Hallelujah!

4:15 p.m.

Another Columbus documentary. When will the makers of these films realize and acknowledge that Christopher Columbus didn't discover anyplace that hadn't been populated, civilized, and highly cultured for millennia, nor did he find anything that was lost? Such glory for navigational error and colonial greed!

Monday, February 10, 1992 — 8 a.m. Day 4

With my arms out, hands above my head, I awoke after a restful sleep in a position I haven't been able to assume for years without cortisone!

Today is the fourth day of my fast. According to my reading, a process called autolysis begins soon in which all morbid accumulations such as tumors, abscesses, damaged tissues, fat deposits, etc. are burned or digested and their components re-used or excreted. Is it possible that the nodules on various parts of my body, and the material that fuses the second joint of my left baby finger in a permanently bent position, will also be eliminated? The deposits that clog my shoulders and limit my range of motion? The spurs on my soles?

I'm feeling only slight general pain and stiffness but no particular pain except in my right wrist. Except for one vicious stab now and then, my headache is gone. I'm not especially hungry.

My mind races and plots. My old world, mostly closed to me for so many years, will open much wider if this effort works and I'm able to sustain this miraculous improvement. I'll again be free to do physical work. I'll personally be able to ready my house for sale rather than having to hire someone to do it for me. I'll be able to comfortably move to California!!

Friday, February 14, 1992

I'm breaking my fast today. I can't believe how much better
I feel after seven days without solid food.

Breaking a fast is at least as important as the fast itself, I've
read. Most of the experts agree that it should be done slowly
and carefully, but they differ on specifics such as the number
of days needed to return to new improved 'normal' eating.
Some say it should take the same number of days as the fast
itself while others say to should take half that number and still
others suggest that twice that number is most appropriate.
Some say only one food should be eaten at a sitting; some say
only raw foods should be eaten at first and quickly-cooked
foods added slowly, for example.

Today I'll have a quarter of a small apple for breakfast, a
leaf of romaine—plain—for lunch, and a small micro-waved
carrot for dinner, in addition to the usual alfalfa and rose-hip
teas. I'll decide this evening or in the morning what I'll eat
tomorrow.

I'm so happy that I did this! I'm nearly pain-free and I
have no stiffness at all—not even in the morning. I do feel a
bit weak, but it's no worse than I might normally feel if I'd
missed only one meal. I can't wait to take my first step toward
California! Kev and Rain can hardly believe the progress
I've made; it seems like a miracle to them too—but we're all
holding our breath to see if the miracle holds, since it seems
too good to be true. None of us says it aloud but we're all
remembering that old caveat that when something seems to
good to be true it usually isn't true.

Saturday, February 29, 1992 — 7:10 a.m.

I'm starting another fast this morning. I did miraculously well
on the first one, which I finished two weeks ago, but I foolishly

failed to follow the suggestions of the pros on breaking my fast so I lost ground almost immediately. On top of that, last week I was very cavalier about eating nightshades and junk food and coffee. Now I'm having severe pain and stiffness again.

This time, when I break my fast, I'll add foods one at a time and carefully note how I feel after each one; I'm already suspicious of grapefruit, almonds, corn products, too much tea, and any kind of onions. I'm also suspicious of eating as often as I do, and of overlapping meals in my stomach.

6:30 p.m.

I'm feeling a bit better already! Could it be that food itself is the problem? Might it be a good idea to fast often and regularly?

Saturday, March 28, 1992

The gains from fasting have held but I'd still like to be more comfortable and stronger without fasting again because I've lost a lot of weight which I'm only slowly regaining. I've looked into homeopathy a little and the underlying principles seem credible to me so I'm going to see a practitioner on Monday.

The basic principles of homeopathy pre-date but are somewhat similar to those that support vaccination and standard allergy treatment. Homeopathy is widely used in Europe, and was popular here in the US for a long time until it was pushed out—but not discredited—by political pressures.

I especially like the fact that homeopathic remedies are never toxic and are chosen on the basis of *all* of the symptoms, physical and mental and spiritual, that afflict the sufferer.

Hank Pizer in *Guide to the New Medicine: What Works, What Doesn't* writes,

> Contrary to the medical notion—where large doses of drugs are often used—homeopathy developed the concept of potentizing substances by diluting them. Homeopathic remedies are in fact so diluted that they may have no chemical evidence of the healing substance in the solution that is taken by the patient. In other words, to the homeopath—less means more....As one can imagine, homeopathic remedies have been criticized as placebos from the very beginning.
>
> An appeal of homeopathy and of giving very small doses of remedies is that it is extremely safe. In an age in which allopathic medicine has been criticized for its extreme interventions, homeopathy represents a conservative approach to healing. Homeopathy makes a different fundamental distinction between the symptoms, the patient, and the illness. Each individual's symptoms are a unique expression of the disorder in his or her life force and vital energy....Because of this, (one person) with asthma may receive a remedy that...is for symptoms that are aggravated by cold, accompanied by thirst and aggravated tensions, while another asthmatic will receive a remedy based on fatigue in the morning, a ready tendency to sweat, and the avoidance of food.

Homeopathy never treats a heart, or a joint, or a bladder infection. In fact, it doesn't diagnose and label syndromes in the way allopathic medicine does. Instead, it addresses an entire suffering person, holistically. The homeopathic method is to administer a infinitesimal and specially prepared dose of a material which would cause, if administered in a very large amount, the very symptoms the patient is experiencing. "Like cures like," they say.

In *The Other Medicines* Richard Grossman writes,

...the law of similars is not new. Over 2300 years ago
Hippocrates wrote, "Through the like, disease is produced,
and through the application of the like, it is cured." This
principle was echoed again in the writings of the fifteenth-
century physician Paracelsus, who described the value of
using similars in healing by writing, "You bring together
the same anatomy of the herbs and the same anatomy of
the illness into one order. This simile gives you the
understanding of the way in which you shall heal."

The way in which homeopathic remedies were discovered
is fascinating. Grossman writes,

...doses of animal, vegetable, and mineral substances were
given to healthy people for a period of two weeks to two
months, and the symptoms generated...were carefully
recorded in the exact words of the experimenters....
Over the past 175 years, a compendium has been amassed
that describes the toxic, symptomatic effects of over two
thousand substances and the system of provings (from the
German word prüfung, "test" or "trial") continues to this
day in the homeopathic community. As in the standard
double-blind method used in conventional pharmacological
investigation, about half the test group are used as
"controls," being given an unmedicated placebo. The
materials involved range, in the vegetable category, for
instance, from simple common plants like onions and
St. John's wort to rare species like hemp and wild indigo;
a vast array of minerals, including familiar ones like gold,
copper, mercury, and sulphur, and less common varieties
such as borax, cadmium, and nitric acid; among the animal
species employed, the common honeybee, toads, a variety
of spiders, wasps, and even rattlesnakes provide the basic
ingredients of the homeopathic remedies. (Incidentally, in
all the years that provings have been the central part of

homeopathic pharmacological research, there is no recorded instance of ongoing distress or eventual harm to the experimenter.)

I like the fact that homeopathic research, unlike conventional research, uses only human subjects; it doesn't use other animals who are not able to consent and much less to report the subjective effects of the material being proven. Another thing I like about homeopathy is the fact that mere removal of symptoms is not considered cure; cure is accepted when the patient becomes not only asymptomatic, but returns fully to wellness and comfort and productivity.

Monday, March 30, 1992

My visit to the homeopathic practitioner was hypochondriac heaven! The visit lasted nearly three hours and left no eyelash undiscussed, no illness unremembered, no scar unparsed. I talked about my surgeries, every prescription medication I've ever taken, every childhood disease and inoculation. I answered questions about my every food preference and aversion, favorite sleeping positions. My moods were discussed in detail as well as my relationships, past and present. Each type of pain I've experienced was noted. The health of my parents and children and extended family was reviewed.

The practitioner listened intently, took copious notes, then asked still more questions. Toward the end of the session, she flipped back and forth between two thick volumes laying open on her desk. She asked a few more questions, flipped back and forth some more, then named the remedy she thought would work for me. She also warned me that I might get worse before I got better.

The remedy she prescribed is rhus toxicodendron. *The Pocket Manual of Homeopathic Materia Medica* by William Boericke, M.D. reads,

> *Rhus Toxicodendron* (Poison ivy)…affects fibrous tissue markedly—joints, tendons, sheaths—aponeurosis, etc., producing pains and stiffness. Post-operative complications. Tearing asunder pains. Motion always "limbers up" the patient, and hence he feels better for a time from a change of position. Ailments from strains, overlifting, getting wet while perspiring. Septic conditions…Rheumatism in the cold season….Face—jaws crack when chewing. Easy dislocation of jaw….Back—Pain and stiffness in small of back; better, motion, or lying on something hard; worse, while sitting. Stiffness of the nape of the neck. Extremities—Hot, painful swelling of joints. Pains tearing in tendons, ligaments, and fasciae. Rheumatic pains spread over a large surface at nape of neck, loins, extremities; better motion….Pain along ulnar nerve. Tearing down thighs….Tenderness about knee-joint. Loss of power in forearm and fingers…

Yep, that's me.

Thursday, April 2, 1992

It worked! It worked! It worked! This is amazing!

I took the remedy as instructed and within hours became much worse. I was in agony for about thirty-six hours and couldn't even sleep off this anticipated exacerbation. After the pain and stiffness finally began to ease, I did drop off to sleep and awoke, eleven hours later, feeling miraculously better.

I cannot believe this! I can't believe that fasting and homeopathy aren't standard treatments for all people with RA;

this is miraculous! Does the Arthritis Foundation know about this?

Tuesday, September 15, 1992

Slouching, belly foremost
scanning the sky
finding nothing there but black cacti
I'll just close my eyes and watch
paisley ladybugs in close
order drill lining my eyelids
smell chlorine and Coppertone and charcoal smoke blowing
off summer
as a myopic ant meanders through my musty sandal
and something not a bird
demands whit to who?

By early April, I was well enough to take my first steps toward California and starting over. The time was definitely right; Kev had decided to make his home in Wisconsin and Rain was as enamored of California as I was, and was certain she would settle there after graduation; neither needed me to maintain a home any longer. I spent the month of April preparing to offer the house for sale.

A realtor listed our place on the first day of May and I accepted an offer on the last day. I spent the week of my fifty-fourth birthday pricing the overwhelming residue of twenty-five years of householding and a fifteen-year collection of back issues of *Writer's Digest* for sale from our garage. I shipped eleven boxes of books and mementoes to Rain in California and, three weeks later, what little hadn't been sold was picked up by Goodwill.

While the buyer of our condo was going through the process of arranging financing, I made my first-ever visit to Kev in Wisconsin; I'd never been well enough to tolerate the trip before. I returned in mid-July to close the sale, hug my brothers and sister and nieces and nephews and friends goodbye and board Continental flight 1003 for San Francisco. What an adventure!

Now I'm getting to know this area and spending time with Rain before classes resume. On the twenty-fourth, I'll be visiting my sister Judy in Tacoma.

These days I'm taking two aspirin a day and nothing else! Even though I'm being very careful of what I eat, I'm a little stiff in the morning, and I have a certain amount of general pain. I can't kneel or run—yet. In fact, I can't walk far at all— but I'm Super Woman compared to the way I was for so long. I want more improvement but I can settle, with gratitude, if this is it.

Monday, November 10, 1992

> *Dragging this bag of old bones makes*
> *my joints ache and fire rage*
> *across my shoulders*
> *down my spine—my own cross.*
> *I should assay them I've heard*
> *old bones are priceless like old books and pressed flowers.*
> *I hesitate.*
> *Its contents might be worthless*
> *then I'd have to drag*
> *an empty bag.*

I awoke with much shoulder and neck pain, and limitation of shoulder, arm, wrist, hand, finger movement. I took a homeopathic remedy and an hour later two aspirin. By noon the pain was greatly reduced and my fingers were much more flexible and comfortable.

I've been slowly losing ground and I can't figure out why; I've been very careful of what I've been eating. Maybe the problem is lack of exercise; I've been depressed by the overcast weather so I've been spending much of my free time reading indoors. I'll make a definite effort to get more exercise even if it's just walking up and down the halls at work.

Tuesday, December 22, 1992 — Happy Solstice!

Fall here was confusing. It smelled like fall, and temperatures "tumbled" into the sixties, but there were only twelve red leaves and seven yellow ones blowing around with about a million crisp green ones! I feel deprived that I can't find a real McIntosh apple—a *Michigan* McIntosh—anywhere; and I just barely made it through late summer without Michigan strawberries and cantaloupe.

We've finally had some rain over the past two weeks and this afternoon we had about five minutes of hail in sixty-degree weather! My neighbor has brought in a fresh Christmas tree so now the house smells just right for the season but it certainly doesn't look right. Inside the glass wall stands The Tree in all its traditional decorated glory; outside that same glass wall, instead of the cold white winter wonderland to which I've been conditioned since childhood, rhododendrons bloom, and azaleas, lemons, oranges, tangerines, and Christmas cacti.

Monday, January 4, 1993

A perfectly functional IBM 286 clone waits a few steps away
but somehow I can't bear to use it to record such thoughts
as I'm having now while an almost-full moon rides high in a
clear cold sky glittered with stars. I'm sad because I don't see
that our beautiful planet can survive our human stewardship
much longer.

I step outside my room (I'm grateful that it's built directly
upon the earth and not elevated above it or above a basement)
into cold air too heavy with the seductive smoke of too many
romantic, decorative wood fires in too many local fireplaces. A
cozy smell, a primitive smell, a smell of home, hearth, evening.
But too many, too much, too long, too often—like most of the
things we do—causing too much degradation of the air we all
need to breathe.

I'm reading *In the Absence of the Sacred,* by Jerry Mander,
in which he details the horrors of unbridled technology and
personal greed. He reports how native Americans and other
indigenous peoples have been tricked out of lands and decent
lives and into slavery to a treadmill they can't escape. This
makes me angry but I see it's not only native peoples who have
been tricked and enslaved; it's everyone, especially the most
sophisticated who, like native peoples knowing not what they
have done to themselves and their children, are no less gullible
or naive.

Most Americans, especially the most prosperous, collude
in an elaborate game of "The Emperor's New Clothes."
I don't *believe* that most people truly enjoy having cash
production by the clock and calendar as the centerpieces of
their lives. I don't *believe* that most people, even those who do
enjoy the work they do for cash, truly want to do that work
for forty—and how much less for fifty or sixty or more—
hours per week for fifty weeks per year for all the forty-plus

years between school and retirement at age sixty-five or seventy. I don't *believe* that most people even truly want or enjoy what they are able to purchase with their labor.

Land use is a *birthright* of *every* creature *regardless* of what all the governments of time and place decree. Each creature should have use of enough land to live upon and glean a living from but no one should own land and no one person should amass land for empire. No one person should control unused land. No one should block access to natural attractions— beaches, mountains, desert—thus all occupied lands should be surrounded on all sides by public lands of passage and sanctuary. Land could be claimed by proxy when a child is born and used for the benefit of the child until she assumes stewardship but when someone dies no land use claim should survive.

Basic to reclaiming a decent way of life is acknowledging that we are indeed all children of this glorious dirt from which we've been so unwittingly alienated by such ambitious devices of history as the notion that homo sapiens is the masterpiece of a sappy god heavy into hierarchy and sado-masochism. Or that dirt, the soil of the earth, is unclean; or that dominion over "lesser creatures" is man's; that man has a mission to increase, multiply, amass, divide, conquer, profit, and to harness Nature and deliver it from its earthy processes of birth, procreation, and death.

Worst of all are the lies that there is no private resonance with the cosmos, that the obvious evolution of the earth can't be trusted and that man's white-knuckled precocity, which delivers misery and death to the individual, will magically bring heaven to earth if only he does it long enough and hard enough.

We forget that we are children of the earth because we were born and have always lived on the platforms in space which we call buildings. We see ourselves *above* all of nature in a literal way as well as a philosophical way. Our food comes un-soiled and glistening with wax or plastic from gleaming supermarkets. Even our corpses are euphemistically returned to the earth sheathed in taffeta, polyfoam, metal, and waterproof concrete; our bodies could last longer in death than they did in life. Even our wanted babies are harvested from engineered, approved, managed, medicated, monitored, draped pregnancies; only unwanted babies come from musk and earth and the barefoot passions of love, lust, or desperation.

Living upon these innumerable platforms, without conscious memory or conviction of a need for land from which to gather food and, foremost, upon which to set feet or lay down to rest, homeless people become schizophrenic and schizophrenic people become homeless. The landed war with the unlanded yet, when a ranking of human needs is expressed, those listed first are air, water, food, clothing, shelter; never listed is the need for *place.* Yet, without satisfying this most elemental need even the most overfed, well-dressed, best-housed and propertied billionaire has no more basic security on his great ornate platform than a single mother on her tiny one. Both *rent* their places on this planet day-to-day from the mob and when the fortune of either is lost, so is any recognized right to even a square inch on which to stand *en pointe.*

Still, the call of Earth is strong. For many people, a vacation must include some form of getting closer to Earth— off-the-grid cabin, tent-camping, sleeping under the stars if not living outdoors altogether. We go where weather permits minimal clothing for maximum skin contact with air and elements. We move closer to other animal species, at zoos, sanctuaries, farms, in the wilderness. Stylized dining is replaced by cooking over open fires then lingering with the smoke, the falling dew and darkness, the night sounds of earth.

Many men participate in seasonal rituals of hunting for game or fish, and some routinely provide meat for their tables in that ancient way, yet what many of them speak of is less the thrill of the chase and the promise of quarry and more of the peace and calm they find in sitting alone in a blind or a boat, observing the energy and intelligence of other animals, the silence of the earth. Some grow beards and gaze into fires and commune with their dogs and each other in ways that sometimes become scary and often must be brought back under control with alcohol and other drugs, carousing, or general machismo.

Hunting or vacationing, or going home to the farm, most people return to captivity refreshed, renewed, relaxed and reluctant to step back into harness. Often the explanation for this reluctance is that man's fallen nature makes him lazy and irresponsible and, if he is not allowed these periods of escape and indulgent delinquency, he will rebel entirely.

Well, part of that is true; for only so long can Nature's whispers be masked by the white noise of this spinning artificial reality that keeps us all moving at top speed and utterly disoriented. But it is not into weak-kneed indulgence that we fall; in fact, we leap instinctively into the very laps of the gods themselves.

Wednesday, January 6, 1993

Compared to this time last year, I'm still doing very well, but my RA symptoms have been gradually worsening over the last months so I consulted a new homeopath yesterday. She gave me a dose of *causticum* and now I'm much worse; I assume this is a predictable aggravation, the phenomenon of getting worse before getting better, which even orthodox medicine recognizes. If so, the symptoms should subside before long and I should improve after that.

Tuesday, January 19, 1993

Finally! Literally overnight, I'm suddenly better after sleeping an unaccustomed twelve hours. I've been needing six aspirin almost every day and I've been terrified that I was having a full-blown relapse.

Saturday, January 30, 1993

This is officially the rainy season but today was wonderfully sunny so I spent several hours outside. This is the sixth year of drought here. Coming from a place called the Water Winter Wonderland, I can't fully appreciate yet how it is to be uncertain of not which day but which year will bring the next rainfall. Conserving water is an utterly foreign concept to me but I am working at taking shorter showers, not letting the water run while I brush my teeth, washing vegetables in a bowl of water rather than under running water.

Rain and I went to see the Kodo Taiko Drummers from Japan. What a thrill it must be to have and use such powerful bodies in such a beautiful way!

Monday, February 22, 1993

I had my follow-up appointment this afternoon. My improvement is holding so the appropriate treatment is to do nothing further until there is another change. It seems weird that homeopathy advocates taking the medication only until improvement begins whereas standard medicine says "finish the prescription."

This morning I planted strawberries and chives at the foot of the tangerine tree while chatting with my old friend Dawn. She'd spent the past week visiting her daughter and mother in the central valley, and the morning here with me on her way back to the airport in South San Francisco. Even though I'd told her in letters about the improvements in my health, she was incredulous about how close to normal I am now; we talked about the days when our visits were mostly at my house because it was just too difficult and painful for me to share in the other usual things friends do together.

This evening I watched Bill Moyers' *Healing And The Mind* on PBS. I've been convinced for years that the mental, emotional, and spiritual aspects of this disease—and maybe any disease—are perhaps even more important than the purely physical aspect (as if there is a dividing live there somewhere…). Since our culture unquestioningly accepts the primacy of the physical, however, to speak and act otherwise is still to swim against the current. Since I was soundly chastised many years ago by my first rheumatologist after I told him that, in addition to the gold salts injections he was administering, I was using the imaging and meditative techniques described in Simonton's and Matthews' book, *Getting Well Again,* I don't often acknowledge this conviction.

Saturday, March 13, 1993

March grass spikes too shy
to burst into green
brilliance in the dew,
clipped into stocky germanic conformity
beyond my curtains, beyond my shade, beyond my window
pilgrims passing.

A warm overcast day in which I had a most mysterious and wonderful experience. For about one hour this afternoon, I had absolutely *no* pain, *no* discomfort, *no* limit to my range of motion—*none!* I felt as if I'd had a cortisone injection—but without the unpleasant side-effects.

This evening, however delightful that magic hour was this afternoon, I'm back to a livable degree of pain and stiffness, but I have even more hope now for a complete recovery. I suppose the explanation for my miraculous experience is that something, somehow, triggered a release of endorphins. In any event, I'll take it and hope for more!

Thursday, March 18, 1993

*Contemplative pines
meet the coming of darkness
with soft spring candles.*

This evening Rain and I are going to see *Indochine.* I love going to the movies and each time we go I vow to go every week—although I've never quite made it. I'm still giddy as a child with my new comfort; I appreciate the movies so much since for so many years I couldn't tolerate the pain and stiffness that would result from sitting in one spot for the length of a movie.

Sunday, May 9, 1993 — Mothers' Day

Rain and I spent a good part of the day at the annual Stanford powwow. Although I'd been to fieldhouse powwows at the University of Michigan and at Eastern Michigan University, I'd never before been to one that was held outdoors. It was quite a different experience although the traditional elements are

always the same, circles within circles within circles. The
drum is always the inner circle—although the drum is in fact
usually a series of drums, each with several players, located at
different spots around the next circle, the dance ground. The
dancers are the next circle, then the spectators. The outer circle
includes the traders and food service, and the final circle is the
campground.

Grand Entry is always indeed that. As the dancers process
slowly onto the dance ground and move clockwise around
the circle, it's easiest then to study and appreciate the details
of the traditional regalia worn by each dancer. Later, during
traditional dancing and competitions, it's difficult to pick out
individuals and details; I'm usually mesmerized by the whirling
colors and bobbing feathers and flying fringe.

We ate Indian tacos, piñon nut porridge, Indian tea, and
wojapi, a sort of blueberry sauce, like thin pie filling. Rain
bought some silver earrings and I bought a braid of sweetgrass,
a copy of *The American Indian Digest* by George Russell, a book
on finger-weaving and a first book on learning the Cherokee
language. We danced a few inter-tribal dances which, as the
master of ceremonies always explains, are for members of any
tribe from anywhere on Earth. We danced a friendship dance
in which dancers in two concentric circles move in opposite
directions and shake hands with each person as they pass.

I picked up some material on the American Indian
College Fund. I didn't know there was such a thing but, since
there are twenty-nine member schools and 80% of the students
in these schools live below the poverty line, I imagine Indian
college administrations have been putting their funds into
actual education rather than fund-raising. But isn't that kind
of like eating your seed corn?

I'm shocked that I *wasn't* shocked to read in *The American
Indian Digest* an excerpt from the 1991 U.S. Department of

Education report, *Indian Nations At Risk Task Force,* "Our
schools have failed to nurture the intellectual development and
academic performance of many native children, as is evident
from their high dropout rates and negative attitudes toward
school.

"Indian lands and resources are constantly besieged by
outside forces interested in further reducing their original
holdings.

"Political relationships between the tribes and the federal
government fluctuate with the will of this U.S. Congress and
decisions by the courts." So much for solemn treaties.

We stopped at the Indian Health Service booth and I was
appalled that the incidence of diabetes among Indians is 680%
higher than the incidence among non-Indians; tuberculosis is
740% higher; alcoholism 612%, and fetal alcohol syndrome
330%. These figures apply to a community whose average
annual income is $7,000.

But, as Russell writes, "Indians are a durable and
resourceful people. They have survived 400 years of genocide
and 100 years of BIA dominance and government control.
They have a strong spiritual nature closely tied to the land and
their religions reflect a respect for the mysterious powers of
nature.

"For the moment, it appears that the pendulum of social
conscience has swung in favor of Indians. There are people of
conscience who empathize and speak out against the plight
of Indians. In academic circles there are concerted efforts to
include a more accurate account of American Indian history
and culture."

After only a short time with the drumming I feel
recalibrated; my gait and even my heartbeat are slower and
more regular for days afterward. I have no words for the way

I feel at a powwow. I've known people who had never attended one who imagined a powwow as only an occasion for drunkenness, orgiastic dancing and general rowdiness; how surprised they were to learn that a powwow is *primarily* a spiritual ritual and family reunion, and that even the social aspects, such as eating and drinking and buying and selling, are infused with a religious solemnity.

Of course, there's always the dry Indian humor: this year's program features the announcement "No drugs or alcohol allowed. Committees are not responsible for accidents, injury, theft, or short-funded travelers."

Sunday, July 4, 1993

Old dandelion
coarse, scorned, common, puffy, tough
faded, still foppish.

Walking in the park, I was greeted by a very old little man, maybe a hundred years old with huge scarred hands, sitting on a bench, proud and dandy in his pale blue leisure suit and shiny white plastic shoes and belt, tiny paper flag pinned to his lapel—a living, breathing Norman Rockwell diorama.

After all these years of wanting to but being stalled by my fear, I've finally had my ears pierced! I'm bewildered as to why I've had this fear when I was never put off by twelve years of almost weekly blood drawing, and twelve years of injections, and more than twenty combined hours of surgery—counting two Caesarean sections.

Rain and I went to an organ concert at Memorial Church; two grad students played duets and ended with Bach's *Toccata and Fugue*. Wow! Like being inside the instrument.

Friday, August 20, 1993

I'm visiting Kev in Madison this week. It's great to be here amid wide lawns and mile after mile of cornfields and dairy cows. And unpredictable rain. And humidity. Somehow I forgot about humidity. Somehow I forgot that mid-western humidity has the power to throw you into a chair and hold you there for breathless hours at a time.

We spent most of today on the road. We took a tour in a refurbished World War II amphibious vehicle which plied the narrow river gorge and majestic rock formations that are the famous Wisconsin dells, then bounced back onto land to wind through a deep and secluded valley where the light is green and hundreds of varieties of ferns grow under a vaulted canopy of treetops.

We drove to Spring Green and Devil's Lake and fell apart laughing each time we saw another "Start Your Day With Pork" billboard. We stopped at an orchard stand for some early cider whose perfume lured us in, but it was a little too early, I guess, because the cider was flat and sour.

Tuesday, September 1, 1993

Back in hot, dry, sparsely-lawned but ever-luscious northern California, this is home now, I realize. I wish both of my children were here with me among all the beautiful California botanicals, oleander and star jasmine, naked ladies and lilies-of-the-Nile, to celebrate Rain's twenty-first birthday.

My shoulders have been bothering me again. I guess I'm starting to take this better health for granted because I get a little sulky when I'm less well. I do actually forget about RA for periods of time and it's usually my deformed hands and feet, rather than my limitations, that remind me.

Saturday, September 18, 1993

I planted daffodil bulbs this morning and this afternoon a group of us went to a Greenpeace benefit art fair and concert in a field in Pescadero. With acoustic music, tie-died tee-shirts, beads and head-bands, peace signs and beards, it resembled a very mini-Woodstock except that it did seem that most of the grass was firmly attached to the earth.

My shoulders are still bothering me, especially when I use the telephone. I bought a shoulder cradle to hold the receiver and that helped. I realize I've almost forgotten about the handicapper aids I left behind—the button-hooker, zipper-pull, grabbers, doorknob adapters, special knives, stocking pullers, spring-loaded scissors, grippers of various kinds, the speaker-phone I used when my hands and shoulders couldn't tolerate the receiver.

Friday, December 10, 1993

A traditional Christmas concert at Memorial Church has opened the Christmas season for me. I'm surprised to realize that, after almost thirty years away from it, the Catholic church building is still, in my mind, the model for all churches. Without a tabernacle and side altars and statuary, Protestant churches look incomplete, even barren, however beautiful with stained glass, carved wood, and magnificent ceiling and wall art.

I had another appointment with Dr. K. last week but so far I'm not responding to the new remedy; in fact I'm getting worse. But I'm trying to keep in mind how my current health situation compared to my situation before I switched to alternative treatment; I've been, overall, infinitely better for nearly two years.

Monday, December 27, 1993

Kev is here for Christmas break. So far, we've gone to the aquarium at Monterey Bay and up to Muir Woods. We drove down the coast to San Gregorio and while I was bundled in sweats, coat, scarf, and mitts against the beach wind, Rain and Kev waded a few feet into the surf. Ah, youth…

Thursday, January 6, 1994

I don't seem to have gotten any better with the last three homeopathic remedies; in fact, I'm getting worse so I have an appointment with an acupuncturist for tomorrow. I've done enough reading to think she can help and I have some idea of what to expect. I'm relieved to know that the needles are ordinarily left in place for only about half an hour although timing varies with practitioner, as does the size and precise placement of the needles and the number used in any given situation.

So far it sounds as if acupuncture can relieve pain but may not be able to correct the underlying problem. Paul Marcus in *Thorsons Introductory Guide to Acupuncture* writes, "Once rheumatoid arthritis, for example, has caused muscle wasting and bony resorption leading to deformities of the joints, this process is not reversible by acupuncture; nor indeed by any other medical treatment."

Marcus explains, "The aim of all forms of treatment by acupuncture is to stimulate nerves running through the skin, and sometimes in deeper tissues. A small area of inflammation is caused, by mildly damaging the cutaneous tissues, which ensures that the stimulation is long lasting. It follows that any method of causing slight trauma to the skin may be used…"

According to Hank Pizer in *Guide to the New Medicine:
What Works, What Doesn't,*

> Acupuncture has been used for treating the chronic pain of
> arthritis…The simplest acupuncture treatment for arthritis
> involves inserting the needles into points near the affected
> joints. If there is muscle tension around the painful joint,
> this therapy may work by breaking the pain cycle in the
> muscle…
>   Another recently offered explanation…hypothesizes
> that the insertion of the acupuncture needle blocks the
> pain message before it can get to the spinal cord and brain.
>   A third possible explanation for the effect of
> acupuncture in arthritis comes from our newly evolving
> understanding of brain chemistry. In some studies,
> acupuncture has been shown to promote the release of
> endorphins in the brain. These neurochemicals…are the
> most potent pain-relieving substances known.

Leon Chaitow in *The Acupuncture Treatment of Pain* writes,
"The usefulness of treating points distant from a site of pain
has been clinically proved. In certain rheumatic and muscular
conditions, distant points may be treated prior to local points
being used." Chaitow goes on to list twelve meridians, or
energy channels, along which needling may be done; for
example, "The kidney (K) meridian starts on the sole of the
foot. It ascends the medial aspect of the leg and runs up the
front of the abdomen to finish on the thorax, just below the
clavicle…The heart (H) meridian begins in the axilla and runs
down the anteromedial aspect of the arm to end at the root of
the little fingernail (medial aspect)." Sounds impressive but, as
usual, the authorities disagree as to why the treatment works
and how it should be administered. I'm really anxious to try
it even though it doesn't sound wildly promising.

Friday, January 7, 1994

Acupuncture seems almost as miraculous as steroids! My shoulders were much improved after spending only an hour with hair-fine needles bristling from my ankles, wrists, left shoulder, and head. What's especially interesting is that, although only my left shoulder was needled, both shoulders are better. I've scheduled a series of seven appointments over the next ten days.

The process wasn't at all intimidating and didn't hurt at all; in fact, the hour flew by as Mary and I found many things to talk about once she had inserted the needles. After I left the office I felt very relaxed and warm and oddly heavy. I'm looking forward to the next visit.

Tuesday, February 1, 1994

Acupuncture has continued to be effective. My left shoulder had been so painful that it was getting very difficult to do my work so I was amazed that the very first session helped so much to realign the joint and minimize the pain. Mary also gave me a food prescription—a combination of rice, other grains and seeds, a few beans, and some Chinese herbs. Fortunately, it tastes pretty good because I'm supposed to eat it twice each day. I've bought several more books on acupuncture and am trying to deepen my understanding of how it works.

I've decided to continue with acupuncture, since it has definitely helped, after discussing the situation with my homeopathic physician. However, she recommends against combining acupuncture with homeopathy.

I ate quite a few acidic foods yesterday and I think they are the cause of today's fresh pain. Certain plants need a more alkaline diet—perhaps I'm like them. All aerobic plants need full-spectrum light in varying amounts and strengths—could that be true of me?

Saturday, March 12, 1994

This is my sabbath. Quietly writing under a white sun, amid cool breezes and the sounds of girls and boys playing baseball in the schoolyard on the next block, the fragrance of coffee roasting at the café around the corner, helps me to regain my perspective.

Richard Geldard in *The Esoteric Emerson* reminds me to "Marshall energies, choose what to seek, then attend to the crucial moment of awakening." He stresses the Emersonian principle of continual reassessment of ideas in light of the latest revealed laws. I need to corral my energies and specifically choose to express my spirit in writing and to begin to submit my writing for publication. I've done a lot of reasoning about the subject, but not a lot of marshalling of energies that will result in decision and action.

I think now that my RA, a disease of bodily connective tissue, an inadequacy, or weakness, or congestion, or infiltration, or occupation, has symbolized and mirrored the lack or inadequacy or inconsistency of my organizing principle—the connective tissue between body and soul. If this is true, then creating, choosing, strengthening my spiritual organization—through the discipline of writing or any other appropriate regular exercise—will be reflected in my body, will help eliminate RA. And still I hesitate. Why?

Step right up to
be disemboweled by
civilization. Stop.

Stand still while rain
craters punctuate
the writing on the wall.

The line forms here
front to back like spoons
behind lost sheep.

Television news keeps me perplexed about my duty to the
occupied, enslaved, and disenfranchised peoples of the US and
the world. I can't seem to find an appropriate way to look at
social problems so I can figure out what I should be doing
about them but I do believe that all that is necessary for evil to
prevail is for good people to do nothing (Margaret Mead?). So
I do a little, mostly contribute money, but I'm certain I can and
should do more, despite my particular limitations.

Saturday, April 9, 1994

When will I just give up on writing? Maybe today I'll just
finally accept the fact that I'll never be the great American
novelist. A person who would think of keeping a used Earl
Grey decaffeinated tea bag overnight in a glass in the
refrigerator to see if it could be used again the next day
because a tea bag makes more than the single cup she drinks
at a time and it's such a shame to waste anything, especially
in these days of concern for all the waste we humans are
covering and filling the earth with, and who writes such
interminable run-on sentences and who dangles prepositions
so precipitously, undoubtedly lacks the attitude and skills to set

down on paper anything that anyone would invest precious
time on...

Besides that, I'm a Gemini—a communicator, yes, but a
person of two minds, and two wills, neither of which is very
disciplined, so I blow hot and cold about writing anyway.

I blow hottest after a hard week of counting the beans of
the company for which I toil. I want to be retired from the
marketplace, to sit in the shade of a live oak tree halfway up a
golden Sierra foothill, to breathe quietly and oversee the bustle
of younger folk below. With an iced tea at my elbow, a yellow
pad on my lap, I long to write my memoirs and speculations.

I could write the memoirs of a good Catholic girl from
East Detroit who wanted to be a nun yet who ended up as an
agnostic divorced mother accountant still enamored, after all
these years, of Ralph Waldo Emerson and Bob Seger. I could
write the speculations of a feminist who wonders whether we
women took a gravely wrong turn when we followed the
men-folk out into the marketplace instead of convincing them
to come back home to work.

I could speculate that, had they noticed that possibility
at the time, our fore-mothers might have pointed out to each
other and to the men in their lives the exorbitant price of
being able to claim the title *head of family, head of household,
man of the house*—even when his home *was* his castle—was—
and is—very high since it includes having to work too many
hours for too many years, for too little money, too little honor,
too little assurance that today's job will be tomorrow's job.
Since it includes being away from home and family for the
best hours of most of the days of most the weeks of all the
months for nearly a half-century. Since it includes expending
the best energies of most of a lifetime doing the bidding of
others who could not care less whether their plans were agreed

to by the peons carrying out the orders. I could speculate that being a man, under the current dying system, includes all of these elements and still being only a paycheck or two away from being *king of the road.*

Instead of writing my memoirs, however, I sit in my little study, tired from the week, old perhaps, watching through glass as scrub jays frolic in this morning's rain puddles. The golden foothills are a few miles beyond our courtyard and little groups of people dedicated to egalitarian principles, non-violence, and sustainable living and loving practices, are popping up in the mountains and beyond in all directions. These are not scared and white-knuckled survivalists nor blind idealists; they are mostly intelligent, hopeful groups that are trying to cut their losses and the losses of the larger world community. I've read lately of several hundred such groups and surely there are hundreds, if not thousands, more. Oh, well, perhaps another day...

My neighbor left a yellow iris in a juice glass outside my door this morning and smelling it precipitated a flood of memories of the springs of my youth—of May crownings with urns of irises, and lilacs tumbling from vases ranged along the altars. Tulips, too, and fruit blossoms—apple, pear, cherry. Hymns to Mary, the mother of Jesus, in the twilight...soft candles, girls in first communion dresses or prom formals... Mary's crown of violets, rosebuds, and ivy...everything soft, gentle, blurry, feminine. When we rehearsed in the unlighted gym/church the day before, all was shadowy and cold like a basement or a storeroom, but in the evening, with the lights and the candles, it was like Christmas should be—full of grace and glowing...

...Christmas at Grandma Hooper's, before 1947, while
Grandpa was still living and the year they got the bubble-lights
for the tree...oval pictures of the Sacred Heart and the
Immaculate Heart over the piano...Grandma playing *Moonlight
Sonata, Warsaw Concerto, Flight of the Bumblebee,* and boogie-
woogie...dry bread heels and stale crackers, awaiting the next
batch of bread pudding, in the deep drawer of the porcelain
kitchen cabinet...Teaberry gum in Grandma's vanity drawer in
her bedroom with the yellowing shade always down...cleaning
her face with Pond's cold cream, never water...skinny in her
wheel-chair after her left leg had been sacrificed to diabetic
gangrene...Grandpa's garden and gifts of kohlrabi and patty
pan squash...poisonous red berries near the cistern—with so
many grandkids, why did they never get rid of that shrub?...
the cool, echoing drip into the cistern...Aunt Millie's leg
make-up during the war when silk or nylon stockings could
not be bought...Uncle Donny and Aunt Nellie living upstairs,
just children playing house, having sex, and buying baked
goods from the Mills Bakery door-to-door truck...
Wow, I get a lot of mileage out of an iris!

Thursday, April 14, 1994

I had a two-hour session with another acupuncturist, this
one trained at the University of Beijing; the session was
very different from those I had with my American-trained
acupuncturist. She first spent a long time taking my pulse at
many different points along a line of about an inch on the
inside of my wrist. Then she looked at my tongue and asked
me a few questions and explained that since my disease was
of such long standing it would take more than a few visits
to improve my condition and that acupuncture, like most
medicine, works best in the earlier stages of disease. Still,
she does think I can be helped, so I'm encouraged.

Dr. Shi used many more and much longer needles on the back of my body and she heated the needles and me almost to the roasting point with a heat lamp. It's a pretty helpless feeling to be alone in a treatment room, clothed only in a towel, with a back full of dozens of needles getting hotter and hotter; I felt as if I'd grind myself to hamburger if I tried to rise if someone yelled "Fire!" But when the session was over, my shoulder bones had moved back into proper relationship to each other and they and my neck felt normal once again.

Dr. Shi also gave me a bag of Chinese herbs for a tea and explained how to prepare it and told me to drink two cups of it daily until my second appointment next week. She talked to me rather sternly about the atrophy in the muscles in my arms and shoulders, and showed me exercises to do every day.

Later I wondered if she was playing some sort of cruel joke as I examined the contents of the bag and prepared to brew the tea: various pieces of dried plant material, seeds, a couple of things that look like a pet bird's cuttle-bone, several wafer-thin slices of a one-inch diameter tree trunk and a four-inch length of dried snake skin!

This compost yielded, besides a nasty tea, a sludge of mud on the bottom of the pan in which I boiled it. The tea smelled vile and tasted worse; I don't know if I can force myself to take this regularly however helpful it might be.

In *The Other Medicines,* Richard Grossman writes, "Particularly in the case of low back pain, cervical spine problems, bursitis, tendonitis, osteo-arthritis, shoulder pain problems…it has become acceptable, if not common, for patients to be referred by their physicians for acupuncture treatment." Well, whadya know!

Sunday, May 22, 1994

I've resumed my search for my Cherokee roots. I've been to the Menlo Park Latter Day Saints genealogical library and I've familiarized myself with the equipment and types of data bases they have. The Mormon libraries have a colossal collection of genealogical data on Mormons and non-Mormons as well. I've sent for Great-Grandmother Breslin's death certificate to start.

For about four years I've been trying, with little success, to learn how to recover my Cherokee ancestry. I wanted to join the North American Indian Association in Michigan but learned that I was ineligible since I was unsure whether my great-grandmother was an enrolled Cherokee. Now I know how to check that out but I still feel like a member of the Wannabe tribe.

Sunday, May 29, 1994

It's been a peaceful day alone doing laundry and hanging it outside, sweeping the patio and preparing food for the little Memorial Day lunch I'm having tomorrow, the first entertaining I've done in years.

I completed literacy tutor training on Friday and I'm looking forward to actually, concretely sharing something of what I have with someone who needs and wants it. I can't imagine not being able to read; to me, reading is almost as important as eating. It's the primary way I learn new things and it's my drug of choice when I wish to escape the harsh realities of the world. Obviously, there are other ways to learn and get around the world, witness the staggering number of American adults who are unable to read and write.

Monday, June 6, 1994

I have a literacy student! His name is Andrew and he's a twenty-four-year-old high school dropout who's been working as a picker in a grocery warehouse and has found his limited reading skills are frustrating his hope of getting a better-paying job. He wants to prepare to take the GED examination and seems to be fired-up and ready to work. The literacy program has very limited funding so I bought a GED study guide to use to prepare assignments for Andrew. I'm fired-up too.

Friday, June 17, 1994

Kev was here for six days for Rain's graduation. Graduation week was hectic, like all graduation weeks are, but enjoyable. The weather was too hot for sitting in the stadium so the vendors must have made a real killing selling straw hats, sun block lotion, fans, and cold drinks to those of us who didn't fully anticipate the ferocity of the sun.

On Monday, while Rain was saying goodbye to classmates she might never see again and moving out of the dorm to the house she'll be sharing with two classmates, Kev and I went to the beach so he could see it when the weather was warm. The three of us spent most of Tuesday at the Monterey Bay Aquarium after having brunch with Jim and Elisabeth and Linda in Carmel. We went to Coyote Point and Point Lobos and one evening Kev downed the traditional 'sake bomb' with his sushi at Miyake's. He left yesterday to return to Madison.

Both children have gently but firmly made it clear that they no longer wish to be actively parented. Ah, the end of yet another era. I'm so glad that we all have good relationships with each other.

A mother bird remembers fledging
but a baby bird cannot imagine maturing
she knows she has matured.
She should be allowed that illusion.
Fledglings do arrive
at a nest of their own
and mother might still be there.

Sunday, July 24, 1994

Andrew's fire seems to be burning low. Out of six appointments, he called to cancel two and didn't show up for two. I'm frustrated and feel as if I'm spinning my wheels. I have a new empathy for teachers now.

Rain roller-bladed ahead while I walked the asphalt paths in the baylands for over an hour. I could have walked longer but the wind was getting pretty stiff and Rain was getting sick from the heat. Quite an improvement since the first time I visited the baylands about a year ago and was only able to walk for less than twenty minutes, and then was in joint agony for two days afterward.

I rejoice daily that my health has been so much better for so long, even though I'm still having some problems with my joints. My right knee is worst—egad!—is it flashing back on my famous Soup Fall?

Still I suspect my diet—particularly beans, wheat, lemon juice, fruit, sesame sticks, peanut butter. I'm also suspicious of food quantities. I definitely seem to feel better on days when I eat little food, which isn't often; I'm always hungry even when I'm eating a lot. Why am I so inconsistent about avoiding foods that seem to cause problems? I should stop procrastinating, get organized and figure this out.

Even with what remains of my RA, I like my life as it is, except for one thing. With so many problems in the world, and so many people—the majority?—whose most minimal needs for place, clean water, food, dry and warm shelter, and work are not being met, and who are dominated, persecuted, terrorized, and enslaved on top of all that deprivation, I don't feel right in just relaxing into my comfortable life. It even seems shameful that I have the luxury of time to comfortably consider such things as social justice.

Even though my life is not without its deprivations and injustices, and members of my class are frequently enslaved and brutalized, at least we are, as a group, well-fed and well-clothed, and most of us have warm and secure places of refuge to which we can retire when we're wounded, in which we can usually sleep safely when we're tired, and in which we can plan and dream in comfortable privacy. I need to find a substantial way to share this simple wealth before I can relax in it.

Saturday, July 30, 1994

Twilight. The best time of day even though sirens wail up and down Alma Street. Two hummingbirds engage in noisy aerobatics, exchanging clicking sounds. Scrub jays perch in the oak and warn each other, "Cat! Cat! Cat!," of the innocent tortoise shell cat in ecstatic oblivion under the spell of the grooming comb in my hand.

I'm trying to burn some very dry sweetgrass but it won't catch. Only a thin wisp of smoke wafts toward me until the wooden kitchen match dies; then all I have is a braid of sweetgrass with a charred end. Finally it catches, glows over my bowl of beach sand, and I sweep the smoke toward me in the growing darkness, as my ancestors blessed and cleansed themselves and each other, with the smoke of sweetgrass and

sage. I want something from the smoke and the twilight, but
I can't name what it is.

Tuesday, August 2, 1994

Leggy mother-in-law's
tongue peers through a gloomy
window, hopes
for a grown child's call.

After several hours today spent shopping for clothing I
hereby renew, with full faith and vigor, my declarations that
full-length mirrors are an abomination and that shopping for
clothing is a heinous chore.

Blithe in my unmirrored oblivion, I labor for many
months at a time under the delusion that I haven't changed
much over the years. Then I go shopping for clothing and
I'm forced to notice and accept the fact that the southbound
direction of my fleshy parts is not premature aging; it's just
aging. And I can't quite get a grip on how I feel about that.

If life is a rose, I'm well beyond the full-bloom stage
and the question is whether I will discolor and fall slowly
or quickly apart, shrivel grotesquely into a dry little knot, or
delicately desiccate on the stem until the day the tiniest puff
of air blows my parts to eternity. Am I speaking of my body
or my mind or both?

I don't think I'm most concerned about my mind because
it seems to be sucking up nutrients, ideas and information, at
a greater than ever rate. And retaining more now that I'm no
longer stupefied with massive amounts of aspirin. It's my body
that seems to be losing ground and my heart that isn't quiet.

I am the sponge
rich
heavy
succulent
absorbed of other waters
occupado
discontent.

Saturday, August 6, 1994

Rain and I walked in the baylands again. I was able to walk
farther than ever but we didn't stay long because the heat was
too intense; it was the hottest day so far this summer.

It seems to me that the biggest problem on earth, which
strikes me as a developmental phase through which most
individuals and most cultures must pass, is that virtually
everyone, at least for some brief time, buys the materialist
idea that profit, greed, exploitation, and endless growth are
inevitable—including and especially the exploited. I think
there are situations, including my own at times, in which
blame must be shared by victims who often consent to,
collaborate in, and risk their own victimization by gambling
that *they* will become the ones who end up, in due time, on
top of the adversarial pile.

Thursday, September 22, 1994

I'm sad because Andrew dropped out of the literacy program;
he's being required to work so much overtime that he feels
he hasn't the time to study or to get together with a tutor.
We didn't accomplish much of anything over these three-plus
months, I'm afraid, but he's such an energetic and enthusiastic
young man, the same age as Kev, and is so handicapped by his

poor reading skills, that he'll probably try again—I hope. He said next time he wants to practice on hot rod and rock music magazines instead of the GED study guide. The program director said she'll assign another student soon.

I'm having trouble sleeping again due to pains in my knees, calves, hands, wrists. My shoulder bones seem to be rubbing together with no cushion at all. My knee parts are still slipping in and out.

I've been working too much all summer and spending too little time outdoors and no time writing.

Monday, November 7, 1994

Overheard while waiting in line at the supermarket...

I wanted to be a teacher but
there's an over-excess of them so
I got a job in a shop I
figgered
what the hell...

I have a new literacy student. She's forty, single, has no children and works as a custodian at an elementary school. She has a stable life and lots of time to study. Her goal is to be able to read stories to her little niece.

My knees are still stiff and painful on stairs, especially while descending, so I don't do much stair-climbing. However, a few weeks ago, on a glorious October Saturday, a group of friends and I scrambled around the steps and trails and rocks at Point Lobos and my discomfort was minimal. Walking on the beach, with or without shoes, is usually uncomfortable and

tiring to my knees (it's worse in dry sand, easier in wet) but I
do it because I love the beach, the wind, the cliffs, the seaweed
streamers washed up in the surf, and because being there feeds
my soul.

I can't lift my arms completely over my head yet from
a standing position although I can do so while lying down.
I often take walks of a half-mile or a mile and my pace
is not totally frustrating to my friends who don't share my
limitations. I haven't tried to ride a bike yet although I'm
eager to do so because I'm still frustrated by the fact that I
was never able to ride the three-speed—all the rage that year—
I received as a birthday gift from my husband just as the disease
began to accelerate.

I can't roller-blade. I can't clog-dance or line dance—
yet. I can't run and I miss running. I always ran everywhere
before I got this disease. The last time I recall running I was
in frantic pursuit of Thor the Mighty Sheltie as he made a
desperate break for the open road of our Farmington Hills
subdivision in 1971. I caught him too! I was a natural-born
sprinter and could go like the wind and outrun boys my own
size and age even as late as age twenty-eight! Rain ran on her
high school cross country and track teams; how I envied her!

At night I have a wonderful recurring dream that I'm
running, effortlessly and for hours and hours, up and down
steep seaside hills in some place I don't recognize, but that
sweet feeling doesn't carry over into my days. During most
days I don't have any strong conviction that I'll ever again be
able to run or that I won't. One step at a time—so to speak—
since I am, after all, a woman of fifty-six summers, and I don't
know what bearing that fact might have on the matter of
being able to run after not having run for more than twenty
years!

Wednesday, November 9, 1994

I'm absolutely positive now that certain of my RA symptoms, as well as other symptoms and discomforts, rise and fall with my eating and avoiding particular foods. A good example is the problem I'm having at the moment with my knees; they feel as though the flesh above them, on the fronts of my thighs, is being separated from the underlying bone. It's a searing, burning pain that I don't feel when I'm sitting perfectly still and that I do feel most acutely when I'm in the act of moving, standing, sitting, or shifting. I know now, after nearly three years of very casual observation, that I get this type of pain after I've eaten a member of the nightshade family; yesterday morning I had a healthy bite of a bagel spread with cream cheese with jalapeño and red chiles.

The reaction usually starts within an hour of my eating one of these foods and lasts for thirty-six to forty-eight hours, depending, I guess, on what else is happening in my digestive tract.

I don't know if this reaction can properly be called an *allergy* to nightshades but I've read that more than three-quarters of people with RA have this sensitivity while the sensitivity in the general population is much lower—around one quarter if I recall correctly.

I seem most sensitive to peppers, less so to tomatoes and eggplant, and even less so to potatoes. I seem occasionally to be able to eat small amounts of the latter three but I seem not to be able to tolerate even minute amounts of any kind of pepper (except black pepper which is not a nightshade). I even react to the tiny amounts of red pepper in mild curries or the cosmetic dusting of cayenne on some deli foods.

Another class of foods to which I have a predictable reaction, although I wouldn't call this an RA symptom, is milk products. If I've eaten some milk product during the day I'm guaranteed to have a certain type of leg cramp, or even a full-blown Charlie horse, as soon as I lie down that night. This situation is easily remedied, however, by taking a tiny pinch (enough to fill two typed capital Os one crystal deep) of ordinary epsom salts completely dissolved in a half-glass of water, either at the time I'm eating the food or at the time I'm experiencing the cramps which are preventing sleep. If I take this after the cramps have started I must walk around for five or ten minutes before going back to bed, but it works every time—and walking around without the epsom salts doesn't work. (I found out the hard way that dosage is critical and too much causes a laxative action!) Most of the time I simply don't eat milk products, or other animal products, for ethical reasons first and for health reasons second.

Other foods to which I seem to be sensitive—that is, I feel RA symptoms when I eat them—are bananas, coffee, yeast breads, more than one piece of fruit daily, head lettuce, orange juice (although I can occasionally eat a whole orange without ill effect), onions, whole wheat (I suspect that it's the germ that's the problem), white mushrooms, peanut butter, sesame seeds, and beans. Not being able to tolerate beans would usually be a serious loss for a vegan, yet I seem to thrive without whole beans, perhaps because I have no problem with frequently eating soybean products such as tofu, miso, soy milk, soy sauce.

It seems that an even greater problem I have with food is quantity. I've always eaten much more than anyone else I know and have always been thin, yet eating my preferred way does not work. When I eat the way I like to eat, I have three large meals and three substantial snacks. I don't gain weight—but I do experience arthritic symptoms.

One of the worse symptoms that develops, after a week or two of consistently improper eating is partial dislocation of my knee and shoulder joints. The feeling is severe grinding pain and a sense that the joint is coming apart. The ends of certain bones visibly protrude from the joint, although not enough to tear the overlying soft tissue, and can actually be moved back into proper position with a slight push, although they usually pop back out again. When I've allowed things to get to this point it's usually necessary to have a treatment or two by my friendly neighborhood acupuncturist.

Sugar is one food that makes me feel horrible in many ways. I experience not joint pain but a general muscular ache and soft-tissue sensitivity to touch if I have more than the equivalent of about three tablespoons of sugar a day. Since I don't use sugar in tea or on cereal or fruit, when I eat sugar it is usually in the form of cookies or candy, my appetite for which is consistent with my appetite for most other foods. I'm always tempted to eat too many double chocolate biscotti, too many bitter chocolate-covered orange jelly candies, or too much chocolate mousse with whipped cream; and when I do I pay dearly.

Saturday, November 19, 1994

A skeleton crew of strawberry plants, new grasses, and mosses in shade pools are giddy with moisture after seven months without rain. A rose bush, confused by the height of the sun and the length of the days, identical with those of early spring, offers up tiny orange-red buds.

It's only three p.m. and already I've lost my sunny spot for the day. The sun's angle is so low these winter days that it sinks below the horizon very early.

Sunday, November 20, 1994

Ahhh! A sunny spot at the courtyard table…two adolescent gray squirrels spiral the grizzled trunk of the oak which canopies the courtyard…pale yellow mums, white azaleas, fuchsia fuchsias, red impatiens, ruby blooms on fat Christmas cacti, green baby lemons camouflaged by same-shade lemon leaves, liquidambar leaves laying in wait for the next cruncher…Maja, a fat gray cat training her eyes and powers on the locked and draped glass door, willing it to ope unto her…

> *I meander, mesmerized*
> *by snakes and shiny objects*
> *like mirrors and coins*
> *when all I want is to sleep warm*
> *and feel blood rush through my soul.*

What is the status of my RA and my health today, almost two years after I took them into my own hands?

My shoulders tense and hunch upwards toward my ears, a most uncomfortable feeling to which I respond by increasing the tension and pulling downward. This relieves the hunching for a few minutes. This is an old familiar feeling but one which I've rarely had, if I recall correctly, since I fasted nearly two years ago.

My neck provides its own discomfort and pain. I imagine that the tendons and ligaments in my neck, weakened by RA, are constantly straining, even while I'm in bed, to support my head and to stay in proper relationship with the tissues of my shoulders, back, and chest.

The spurs on the soles of my feet feel like sharp stones under my skin although I suppose they are in fact mineral deposits of some kind—perhaps uric acid or calcium— surrounded by pockets of fluid. Whatever they are, they hurt when I walk barefoot so shoes do help.

The only shoes I can wear are Keds old-fashioned canvas tie shoes. The problem is that, despite all the medical treatment I've had over the years, all eight small toes have become hammertoes so the toe box in most shoes is too shallow. Another consideration is that metatarsal resectioning has made the ends of those bones unable to withstand the additional pressure that results from any heel higher than five-eighths of an inch. So I have an entire wardrobe of 7EEE Keds in every color available for that width—three pairs of white and two pairs of navy.

Sometimes I feel sorry for myself that I can no longer put together a really attractive outfit, including stylish shoes, perhaps even the three-inch heels I wore to work for many years. I no longer look the total professional in my dark business suits because somehow white sneakers—even new white sneakers or navy sneakers—just aren't the same. And then I catch myself and remember that there were times when I could get no shoe on my swollen feet, and I'm grateful to whatever now helps me to walk, work, heal, and hope for more.

My hands are quite comfortable today although I can see slight inflammation around my knuckles. I have the equivalent of hammertoes on three fingers that are frozen at 90° angles at the first joints above the knuckles. The second joint of my right index finger is frozen at a 45° angle. The joint of my right thumb was fused surgically in 1990 because it was bending backwards a few degrees and I was having difficulty writing; now it doesn't bend at all.

I have two two-inch and a five-inch surgical scar on the top of my left hand/wrist and a six-inch scar on the bottom. I have two two-inch and a five-inch scar on the top of my right hand/wrist and a half-inch scar on my right palm. My wrists are a little sore today.

My left knee is unstable at the moment and a bone on the inside pops painlessly out of the joint when I sit down. It pops back in when I wiggle a little, or a little push usually painlessly reseats it. Although I can't kneel, I can walk up and down stairs, and take relatively long walks without feeling that my knees are coming apart or that they will collapse under me. That's all the bad news.

The good news is I can write and I can type and I can earn my living better than at any time since 1978. I can cook and clean; I can even sew, something I wasn't able to do for quite a few years. My hands look as if they've been through a war, as they have been, but they serve me well and I'm grateful. I can walk and I'm stronger every day. I'm no longer frail in any sense. I'm thankful every day to whatever powers and processes have enabled me to reestablish a more normal life.

Monday, December 7, 1994

A dark and windy morning awaiting rain, a morning suitable only for returning to bed. I think we were meant to hibernate; I sleep longer and harder during the winter.

It has become painfully—or painlessly, rather—obvious to me that the more I do, physically and mentally, the more I'm able to do. Two years ago, when I first moved here, it was a challenge to walk the block from my house to the café on the corner. Before I tried it the first time I feared I would be stranded and unable to get back home; when I actually tried it I made it both ways—and was exhausted for hours. While I did have the energy and strength to do things and go places, I didn't yet have the stamina and leg strength to stand very long or walk very far. That was two years ago.

About eighteen months ago, I first went walking in the baylands to meet the flora and fauna and the winds that blow across the open water near the southern end of San Francisco Bay. We walked less than a quarter-mile and I was sore for days. My knees felt as though they were mortally wounded and it was necessary to swab my entire legs with analgesic creme for several nights in order to sleep.

After the worst of that passed, I walked a little longer each day. Most nights my leg muscles and joints were sore enough that I was awakened several times each night and had to walk around in my room to stretch the muscles in my legs. Sometimes I had to use an analgesic creme to get back to sleep.

When I started seeing Dr. Shi, she was appalled at the muscle atrophy in my back and shoulder muscles. In fact, my reason for seeing her was to correct painfully dislocated shoulder joints. She was able to relieve the shoulder problem but she sternly advised me that I should be exercising my joints daily to extend their range of motion as well as to rebuild muscle mass.

Since then I have tended to be faithful to these exercises when I'm having shoulder joint problems but I make excuses for not doing them when I'm feeling better. Since I work seated at a computer or a desk and even the paper files I work with are light, I haven't made nearly as much improvement in my shoulders and arms as I have gradually made in my legs.

Despite my backsliding, I'm sold on the benefit of regular and appropriate movement because of my own experience and one brief demonstration of the marvelous effectiveness of Feldenkrais exercises. I've also experimented, with gratifying results, with simple movement to music. But, as usual and as with food, I don't always follow through and I'm sometimes disgusted with myself for that.

I'm not doing enough writing these days. If I chose to, I could *write* the book for which I searched after I'd seen a TV news article about successful treatment of other medical conditions with so-called alternative methods, now that I've had such fantastic long-term results.

If I were to write such a book, I'm sure it would be pronounced "merely anecdotal" by any rheumatologist I know. Of course, that's all I *could* write—an anecdote of my *personal* experience and the conclusions I've drawn. It could have no imprimatur from any authority more recognized than one person who has lived with the disease, failed with standard treatment, and succeeded with non-standard treatment. It wouldn't be declared free of doctrinal or factual error by anyone. It couldn't be in the least a scientific report.

I'm certain that, if an average rheumatologist were to read such a book, s/he would quickly declare that, at best, there could be no way of knowing whether my remission was a spontaneous one which occurred in spite of, rather than because of, the "quack" methods I employed. I'm equally certain that this same declaration would never be put forth to discount or dismiss a remission following a course of whatever are today's latest allopathic drugs and therapies, even the experimental ones; I'm certain that such an event would be viewed as one of cause-and-effect by this average rheumatologist.

Thursday, December 22, 1994 — Winter Solstice

Waves boil, froth, roll, break, and chase a pack of seagulls up the beach only for them to rush back again with the salty water as it slips back into the ocean. Around the pale December sun the white sky glows and flows into strong blue, bright even through the fog.

Mist veils the sharp cliffs in the near distance, and fogs those beyond. A balmy Wednesday at San Gregorio beach where only a few people stroll the hard wet sand and a handful of playful loons dive under each breaking wave to bob up triumphant in each next trough. Behind us, across Highway 1, soft green mountains roll and swell in womanly fullness. Beauty above me, beauty below me, beauty all around, as the Native American song goes.

Reluctant to leave the beach, we head back out Highway 84, past rolling acres of empty artichoke fields and pumpkin fields fallowing in the soft day, past weathering family farm buildings, following the twists and curves, hairpins and switchbacks through the mountains, then onto 280 and home to prepare for a pot-luck celebration of Winter Solstice, the longest night of the year, when the seed of the coming spring begins to grow.

Seven p.m., as guests arrive at Rain's house, has a middle-of-the-night feel since darkness fell nearly two hours ago on this shortest day if the year. We help ourselves to potato-collard soup with leeks and garlic, linguine with garbanzo-olive sauce, Caesar salad lush with grated Parmesan and anchovy, delicate cous-cous salad with spring onions and pine nuts, sage bread, strawberry-rhubarb pie, chunks of bittersweet chocolate, sparkling cider and plum wine. Eight people manage to get eight plates, eight glasses, and eight pairs of hands and shoulders and knees around a smallish coffee table. Candles, the only light, flicker and glow while the royal cats, Xochi and Atticus, conspire to acquire people food. All keep vigil for the beginning of Earth's new year.

For me this is also another thanksgiving. I am utterly grateful. Grateful to whatever powers and whichever factors have caused me to return so close to full health. Grateful to whatever lifted me out of chronic pain, fluctuating physical limitation, unpredictability. I'm grateful to the combination of materials, conditions, information, intuition and accidents that has allowed me to live an average life for almost three years. After close to twenty-five years of domination by RA I'm now dominated by feelings of gratitude and appreciation.

Saturday, December 24, 1994

It's Christmas eve and an apricot rose blooms in our courtyard next to a white azalea—an Easter flower in my beloved Michigan—and a huge Christmas cactus, fountain-like, sprays its blooms in a wide red circle, brilliant even in this early light. Several times during the night I was awakened by the staccato of raindrops on the skylight. Winter at its wildest in the South Bay is quite like spring thaw in Michigan in that frequent gentle rains maintain an almost hot-house atmosphere.

I can't decide whether overall climate plays an important part in my new comfort but I am certain that day-to-day changes in weather do affect the way I feel. This is my third winter here but I'm still surprised that, at its worst, temperatures usually bottom out at well above freezing— although my neighbor did frantically cover her citrus trees with bedsheets one evening in 1992 when the weather service predicted a drop into the high twenties overnight.

I do know it's important for me to stay warm although my comfort range is narrow and I easily overheat. It's definitely easier for me to stay within that narrow range in California than in Michigan. Artificial heating is needed less here so super-conditioned indoor air is not the problem it was for me in Michigan where humidified forced-air heat is most common. My place here is heated by hot water coursing through pipes imbedded in the floor and the resulting constant temperature is much more comfortable, to me, than the hot-air-blast-fading-to-cool cycling I've lived with for most of my life.

Humidity rather than heat is usually cited as the primary culprit responsible for summer discomfort. I do know that breathing during August days in southeastern Michigan for the last several years I lived there was almost an exercise in futility. On the other hand, sleeping was deliciously comfortable because I was able to be warm enough without the constraint of much clothing or covering and without the constant muscular tension caused by fluctuating air temperatures. Now, even when the ocean fog climbs over the mountains in the evening, it remains high aloft, so humidity and night-time heat are not often problems here.

I do often wonder just *how* significant the climate change has been to my improvement. A logical test would be to return to Michigan to live during a time when I would expect to be uncomfortable—but I'm not so ready to tempt fate! Northern California and southern Michigan are peers in respect to natural beauty but I miss Michigan's special grandeur. I miss the drama and glory of fall colors, blinding white daytime snow and magic blue nighttime snow, the eerie beauty of acres and miles of leafless trees, and hot summer nights. I don't miss heavy coats, snow boots, gloves, icy driving conditions, ice build-up in parking lots and road shoulders, scraping ice from car windows, filthy roadside snow, salt and sand on slippery walks, thirteen-month winters! I miss summer thunderstorms followed by the scent of ozone in the air and the feeling of catharsis afterwards, the fact and effect of an earth freshly-bathed, but I'm not going to volunteer to deal again, long-term, with the violent punishment of Michigan's inclement weather; I'll visit in the summer.

Saturday, December 31, 1994 — New Year's Eve morning

My spurs are definitely reduced. Is it because of the vitamins I've been taking for the past several days? Or the *calcarea fluorica* I've been taking on and off for a couple of weeks? *The Smart Guide to Homeopathy* reads, "*Calcarea fluorica* (Calcium fluoride) Indications: Joint pain, cysts, varicose veins, poor tooth enamel, bony formations, lumbago. Confirmation: Indecisiveness, fatigue, relaxation of connective tissue. Symptoms improved by: Heat and warm applications, continuation of moving, rubbing. Symptoms aggravated by: During rest and beginning to move, damp or humid weather."

Was it the three acupuncture treatments I've had in the past month? All of the above? I'm inclined to attribute the improvement mostly to the vitamins since their primary benefit, in relation to my problems, is to reduce bony formations. The other two methods address that factor as well as specific joint complaints and my joints are less improved than the spurs. In addition, the 'pump bumps' which have inexplicably risen and fallen on the backs of my Achilles tendons for years, are quickly disappearing as well. Could it be that these spurs and bumps as well as the plates I sometimes feel on my ankles and those that partially band my upper arms, all of which come and go so mysteriously, result from an uneven supply of these vitamins or minerals? Could it be that the effect of using *calcarea fluorica,* without vitamin supplementation, is to enable my body to extract these nutrients from my ordinary diet—assuming my diet contains them in the first place?

My shoulders and neck are a bit better but, although not too painful, along with the arm bands, still annoying. My wrists and hands are more painful and my hands have been hot and somewhat swollen. Since I haven't kept a good record of these shifting patterns of pain and comfort I can't recall when

I've had such hand pain for more than a day. Often, after the disease has been flaring for a longer time, I begin again to record my symptoms to see whether a pattern emerges from my reactions to treatment efforts, but I invariably lose interest after a few days and gradually the recording dissipates as the symptoms subside.

My greatest discomfort these past several days has been the feeling of weakness in my neck, as if it's not capable of staying in proper relationship to my head, shoulders, back, and chest. Every few minutes I become aware that my neck has led my torso in leaning forward from the waist and my neck is straining to hold my head in proper position. So I retract my neck, sit up straight and try to maintain this alignment—but I forget, so I go through this cycle perhaps every five minutes.

I should choose one treatment method to stay with so I can chart my progress a bit more scientifically. Still it's difficult to stay with only one option when results are not immediate and other promising options are easily available. I especially like the idea of homeopathy because it seems to be a truly elegant method of stimulating the body's own defenses as well as a more convenient method than acupuncture which also stimulates the body's defenses.

If I choose homeopathy, I must then choose between working with a practitioner or working with a stack of books. If I choose acupuncture I must work with a practitioner. I can also choose to carefully use any combination that seems appropriate, as I have been doing, with and without practitioners, and always with stacks of books. Purists would protest, of course, but perhaps I'll just stick with the intuitive and eclectic approach that has worked so well so far.

Sunday, January 1, 1995 — New Year's Day

"The death of fear is in doing what you fear to do."
  – *Sequichie Comingdeer*

"Do or do not; there is no try."
  – *Yoda*

"Take no counsel of your fears."
  – *Unknown*

...I remind my body to remember its original coding...
recall how it was before there was any genetic mutation or
environmental damage...remember how it was to be entirely
healthy and strong...remember back, beyond the strongest it's
ever been, to its perfect design...Every day, in every way, I'm
healthier, stronger, more robust. Every day, in every way, I'm
more free of disease, of pain, of worry about health...I tell my
body to recall that it knows how to be perfect and healthy...
recall how it feels to be healthy...

I'm still toying with the idea of putting together an
account of my recovery progress; I've lost track of the number
of times I've gone through the thought process. Each time I
make a trial commitment to the idea of writing my journal as
if I'm writing for another reader I soon lose my nerve; I'm an
accountant, a writer in my dreams, my demons remind me.
But all the while I know that, when I was desperate, I needed
to read an account such as I can write and I'm not the last
person struggling with short-lived or ineffective therapies for
RA. Okay, I'll commit myself once again and I'll be still and
steady in the effort. I hope.

My hands were considerably better when I awoke this morning. My shoulders are better, too, although still hunching a bit, but my neck is worse and my throat feels tight. My spurs and right ankle bumps are noticeably better than yesterday, and infinitely better than pre-1992. On my worst days now, I can put all my weight on my feet and stand for long periods, even though there is still pain.

I'm not certain how many doses of *calcarea fluorica* I took yesterday. I should keep records but, even if I did, I couldn't be certain whether the improvement was due to the *calcarea fluorica* or to the vitamins or to the herbal compound I tried (devil's claw, sarsaparilla root, nettle seed, burdock seed, angelica root, and prickly ash bark) or to some combination of these.

The more I read, the more I'm aware of the concordance between homeopathic remedies and herbal remedies; for example, *The Smart Guide to Homeopathy* says,

> *Hypericum perforatum* (St. John's Wort) Indications: Nerve pain due to trauma, post operative pain, lacerations, toothache, deep needle prick. Confirmation: Excessive pain, tingling, numbness, pains radiate along nerve. Symptoms improved by: Bending head backward. Symptoms aggravated by: Cold, damp, fog, touch.

> *The New Holistic Herbal* says:

> St. John's Wort *(Hypericum perforatum)*....Actions: Anti-inflammatory, astringent, vulnerary, sedative. Indications: Taken internally, St. John's Wort has a sedative and pain reducing effect, which gives it a place in the treatment of neuralgia, anxiety, tension and similar problems....In addition to neuralgic pain, it will ease fibrositis, sciatica, and rheumatic pain. As a lotion, it will speed the healing of wounds and bruises, varicose veins and mild burns. The oil is especially useful for the treatment of sunburn.

I'm reassured that there is agreement between these two schools of thought about the properties of many of the herbs and homeopathic remedies I've checked out.

I can hardly believe there are so many types of alternative medicine; I've read descriptions of osteopathic manipulation, chiropractic, ayurveda, massage and polarity therapies, yoga, psychosynthesis, qi gong, oxygen therapy, water therapy, urine therapy (!), multi-wave oscillator therapy, radiobiology, bee venom and chelation therapies, iridology and reflexology, electromedicine and radionics, music therapy and cymatics and microwave resonance therapy, fever therapy and humor therapy, and the purported miraculous properties of pycnogenols, DMSO (dimethyl sulfoxide), and DHEA (dehydroepiandrosterone). I've seen laundry lists of dozens more.

According to Robert Tisserand, in *Aromatherapy: To Heal and Tend the Body,* "An independent survey of alternative therapies carried out in 1984 revealed that the treatments which people were most satisfied with were relaxation and massage. It is important to remember, when looking at the survey results, that they are not hard success-rate figures, but rather reflect the patient's general degree of satisfaction." According to the table referred to, the percentages of patients satisfied and dissatisfied with various alternative therapies were:

Alternative Therapy	Satisfied	Dissatisfied
Meditation/relaxation	83%	12%
Massage	82%	9%
Psychotherapy	75%	12%
Osteopathy	73%	14%
Herbal Medicine	73%	18%
Chiropractic	69%	19%
Homeopathy	66%	16%
Vitamin/mineral therapy	65%	12%
Acupuncture	50%	47%
Hypnotherapy	43%	50%

Tisserand notes, "It may well be that the therapies which did not score so well, notably acupuncture and homeopathy, have a greater potential to produce more lasting health improvements in serious conditions than massage and relaxation therapy...The two top scorers, however, are therapies which aim to make you feel good immediately."

After reading about aromatherapy, I'm interested in trying it; it sounds promising in the treatment of RA. Tisserand writes that "Some essential oils act as blood cleansers/purifiers. These include angelica root and juniper which...promote the elimination of uric acid and are useful in the treatment of gout and rheumatoid arthritis." He describes a case history in which a woman with RA had weekly sessions for two months in which a mixture of the essential oils of chamomile and rosemary were rubbed into her affected joints; she began to experience a lessening of symptoms after the third visit and ten months from the date of her initial visit, she was still free of RA symptoms.

According to Tisserand, "rosemary is a nervous stimulant, and various different studies have shown that it stimulates heart action, respiration, digestion, kidney function, liver function, gall bladder function, blood circulation, and the adrenal glands. It is in fact the most stimulating of all essential oils…Because of its stimulating effect on blood and lymph flow, especially when applied through the skin, rosemary oil is useful for all kinds of aches and pains." The homeopathic materia medica and my books on conventional herbology agree with these uses and effects. As fascinating as aromatherapy sounds, I don't think this is a good time to add another therapy.

If I were choosing only among the three types of therapy I've used recently, I'd choose homeopathy because I know that continued use of only part of the vitamin B complex can induce a deficiency of other B vitamins since they work synergistically and must be present simultaneously in appropriate ratios, and herbal remedies are less convenient and sometimes slower-acting.

It would probably be more efficient for me to work again with an experienced practitioner but I'd still like to see if I can find my way for myself. Although I realize that it's possible to disorder my case if I choose the wrong remedies, the worst that can happen is that I will lose all the ground I've gained and will have to start again. Since homeopathic remedies are not dangerous in themselves, amateur experimentation with lower potency remedies is not dangerous in the same sense that experimenting with conventional prescription medications or even over-the-counter preparations would be.

Conventional medical drugs work to eliminate symptoms rather than to stimulate the body to respond in an appropriate way, so the total long-term effects, beyond symptom suppression, may not be recognized—particularly by the amateur. Exactly the opposite is true with homeopathy. Symptoms would worsen or change obviously so it would be clear that something, perhaps undesired, was happening.

Even homeopathic remedies, however, I wouldn't consider self-prescribing in any potency higher than 30C or 30X since I've already felt and seen, in myself and others, the power of higher potencies expertly prescribed. In fact, I don't take even the lower potencies without seriously studying the books I already have or new ones I add to my little library in order to be certain I know more than the minimum I need to know. I want to be certain in each situation that the remedy I'm considering is not only *appropriate,* but the *best* one for that specific time. Even though I can't cause serious or long-term damage to myself with an inappropriate remedy, I can cause needless confusion and short-term discomfort.

In my experience, treating RA with alternative methods is not only much more effective but far less expensive. The cost of homeopathic remedies is almost negligible and even consultations are less costly than allopathic consultation. It's most certainly less expensive to my insurance carrier, which continues to accept my monthly premium payments and pays out nothing for the *effective* treatment of my most serious problem, yet stands ready to pay out thousands and thousands if I decide to change to *conventional,* and *ineffectual,* treatment.

I've finally found the clearing house I heard about in '84 or '85; it's called World Research Foundation International Health and Environmental Network. I've subscribed to its publication, *World Research News,* which contains in-depth articles on alternative therapies—some of which sound incredibly bizarre—and a catalog of books, tapes, and library and computer information packets for sale.

Monday, January 2, 1995

Today the lower part of my body is doing quite well. The spurs on my soles and the nodules on my Achilles tendons are noticeably reduced from yesterday. In addition, the plate on the

inside of my right foot has nearly disappeared. Although at
times, months ago, this plate hurt as I put my weight on it in
the same way that the spurs on my metatarsal arch hurt, the
pain stopped awhile ago even though the plate was still there.
Now it's being resorbed.

I'm hoping the same thing will happen with the material
that has filled the joints and fused my toes into hammertoes,
and has likewise fused several of my fingers. While these are
not particularly painful, the deformity itself is difficult to deal
with.

My upper body is less well today. Although my hands
and wrists are better than yesterday, my neck still feels as if
it's straining. I wonder if the ligaments and tendons in my
neck and shoulders and upper arms are all weakened by some
additional pathogen. I'm encouraged by knowing that the
homeopathic remedies I'm taking, assuming they are the
appropriate ones, will do their work of stimulating my body's
own defenses whether the pathogens are identified or not.
But I'm impatient for it to work NOW!

One of my goals this year, through medication and
exercise, is to strengthen my knees enough to be able to take a
tub bath and then kneel to clean the tub afterward—not such
a lofty ambition, but I haven't been able to do that since 1982
when I nearly tore the plumbing out of the wall by using it to
pull myself up out of my last tub bath! In my case, the *knees*
were the first to go, to paraphrase the cliché. Right now, I
couldn't even use my shoulders to use grab bars to pull myself
up—so all my parts must heal! Ever since my 1992 experience
of a hot tub in Sparrow Hawk Village, under a million
Oklahoma stars, I have lusted after the experience of again
and often easing myself into the sheer comfort and delicious
pleasure and relaxation of an ordinary bathtub of warm water!

I've rubbed analgesic creme into my neck and shoulders and it's helping a little but the discomfort is still distracting. I must change my position slightly every minute or so to relieve the feeling of fatigue that so quickly develops.

RA has changed from a debilitating disease to an annoying one now that I no longer fear that I'll be unable to function well enough to sustain my life. I came close enough to the profound debility I feared; for years I felt as if I were living on the brink of disaster. Now it's difficult to recall the terror of not being certain—as certain as anyone can be—that I would be able to take care of myself and meet my commitments to my children. Now, annoyed or not, forgetful or not, I'm grateful daily that I've found a way to escape so much limitation and pain and to find so much restoration and comfort.

It's as if I'd been living in a labyrinthine cave that has finally opened into a clear, straight tunnel with a light, however faint and distant, at the far end. While I was in the dark part of the cave I could occasionally see a spark but as I tried to move toward it, through medications and surgeries, it disappeared.

In the beginning, the cave was only cool and dark and damp. Then shockingly quickly, the cave turned frigid and very black, and I was walking in water I couldn't see, and I didn't know whether I'd have to begin swimming with the next step. I could hear shouted instructions from my would-be rescuers, my physicians, but the directions and assurances they were shouting were wrong! They were *wrong!*

And the cave got darker yet, colder, wetter and—terror!— my body responded less and less and my rescuers shouted instructions that were ever more guesses, shots-in-the-dark, experimental combinations of old and new ideas.

After a point, when I realized that the instructions themselves were threatening, I decided I might have greater success by listening to other fainter voices coming from other directions. I listened, I considered, I took a small test step and found myself on slightly higher ground, then another tiny step. Still terrified at each step, I heard the conflicting louder and softer voices, each threatening disaster if I followed the direction of the other.

In the end I could only choose to try each in order and I had already followed the loud voice for a long time; now I would continue to follow the softer and watch for results.

Following the softer voice I've gotten closer and closer to the light. Now I'm in a smooth glass tunnel whose surface reflects the light at its end. My steps are still small and slow because the reflective surface of this portion of the tunnel can also give false impressions, exaggerations, blinding glare. Some of my steps lead backward; on some I don't follow through.

Perhaps my damaged body will never carry me entirely outside the tunnel but each day I do get closer and my body does get stronger, more normal. Even if I don't make it all the way, compared to the way I've had to live for so long, this is fine. Just fine.

Saturday, January 7, 1995

At work this week we dove into year-end closing and overtime. Fortunately, my neck is a bit better and so is my left shoulder and so are my hands, wrists, fingers, and feet! Was it the *calcarea fluorica?* Was it the vitamins? Was it the herbs? Was it my talking to my body? Was it meditation? Was it prayer? I don't know which therapy or combination of therapies would work to cause further improvement so, as in the case of most decisions in my or anyone's life, I'll have to make a decision on the basis of inadequate information.

I imagine that a series of acupuncture treatments might work again to correct the partial dislocation of my left shoulder as it did just about a year ago, but I don't want to commit myself to the time or expense that would entail unless all else that is more convenient fails. For the same reason, I don't want to commit to treatment by a homeopathic practitioner. So I guess I've made the choice, again, to continue treating myself, at least for awhile. I am aware of the wisdom in the words "Who represents himself at court has a fool for a client" but....Again I choose the methods I know most about, diet and homeopathy, and commit myself to learn more. Maybe I'll add more herbs later.

Diet is the easiest to address. For the past six or so weeks, beginning around Thanksgiving, I've too often eaten foods which I know cause problems for me. I've often indulged in a double-decaf-whole-milk latte at the neighborhood café where every afternoon at about two the aroma of the roasting of the beans seduces me yet again to walk zombie-like to pay homage to my coffee god. I don't resist even though I know that milk is a problem for me and that, in drinking even decaffeinated coffee, I'm also risking antidoting the homeopathic remedy I've been taking.

On top of that, I've also had the occasional cup of home-brewed decaf at the homes and offices of others. I've eaten roast pork loin with apples and onions, Spinach Benedict, Caesar salad, Death-By-Chocolate cheesecake, and quesadillas made even more threatening with bits of jalapeño. I've eaten in restaurants where the chile is a staple, in Szechwan food, and Mexican, Thai, Indian food. I've eaten potatoes in the potato-collard soup I made for our Winter Solstice potluck, and in Indian curries, and garlic mashed potatoes at the company's holiday dinner (along with the turkey and trimmings). I've eaten baba ghanouj, a wonderful dip made of eggplant, garlic, olive oil and spices. I've eaten braised eggplant with garlic, and angel hair pomodori with sun-dried tomatoes. Sometimes the food is worth the reaction; often it's not.

I've eaten onions, white mushrooms, yeast breads, and too much fruit, all of which cause an increase in pain and stiffness within an hour or so after eating them. And I've eaten a ton of sweets—cookies, fruit breads, cakes, and chocolate—at work, at parties, at home. I'm addicted to chocolate and several times a day I set out on a search through the office for signs of chocolate. Sweets seem not to affect my joints particularly but, instead cause a feeling of general pain and substantial stiffness throughout my body as well as a general sense of unwellness.

Taken all together, these foods may have caused the flare I'm experiencing now, and apparently the herbs and homeopathic remedies haven't been able to keep up.

Friday, January 13, 1995

The W-2s and 1099s are finally balanced so we'll print them out on Monday and get on with the rest of the year-end stuff. I'm challenged by the need to finalize so much data in just a few weeks but I'm distracted by pain so I'm not enjoying it much.

I can't figure out what's happening. My hands and wrists, especially my right wrist, are worse—worse than they've been in years if I'm remembering correctly. My shoulders, especially the left, continue to be bad despite the homeopathic remedy and recent careful diet. My front thigh muscles feel as if they're being peeled off my bones, the bands around my upper arms feel tight as tourniquets. My thumbs throb. There's an itchy pain at the 'knob' of my neck and at the base of my spine. My neck, shoulders, and back are all crunchy with crepitus. Even the pressure of a chair on the backs of my thighs is uncomfortable. Only my foot spurs are better and my toes are bunching less. My sinuses and eyes are dry. I've been having headaches. I'm miserable.

Monday, January 16, 1995

Like Eve before me, I picked fruit from a tree in our backyard and lived to regret it. I ate a tangerine yesterday and one the day before. This morning I awoke with the spurs on the bottoms of my feet much worse again and an old familiar ache and a new nodule on my right Achilles tendon. I *know* this is a cause/effect situation. I do seem to be able to get away with eating an *occasional* orange or tangerine, or some vegan avgolemono soup, but it does seem that the second serving is more than my body can handle. In recent readings, I've been reminded that now even some mainstream doctors believe people with RA should largely avoid the acidic foods I crave. Before I was told to eliminate acidic foods, and my spurs were so bad that I had to cushion them with moleskin, bunion pads, and thick socks, I was eating one or two grapefruits daily and, next to salt, lemon juice was my favorite seasoning.

Wednesday, January 25, 1995

One of the best things I've ever done for myself was to negotiate my four-day job—although I never realized such things were possible before I came to California. Not working on Wednesdays makes my job seem only part-time; I never work more than two days in a row before I have at least one day to devote to other things. Everyone should work this way! I also never thought of working in the casual attire that's so common here. How could I ever revert to power suits and a nine-to-five five-day work week?

In *The Care of the Soul,* Thomas Moore, in the chapter entitled "The Body's Politics of Illness," writes about taking symptoms out of the realm of chemistry and treating them as symbols. James Hillman and Robert Sardello, according to Moore, "suggest that it is the function of the body to give us emotions and images proper to its highly articulated organs." According to Sardello, "the object of therapeutic treatment is to return imagination to the things that have only become physical." I don't know about anyone else with this disease, but I'm certain that my RA is *both* real and symbolic.

...Drawn by the buzz of the chain-saw, above the housetops a block over, I see a palm tree being dismembered by a worker in a cherry-picker. There are only two fronds left and I see dark blotches where the others have been. Am I witness to cosmetic surgery, murder, or euthanasia?

...Now all its fronds are gone and it stands naked, looking like a giant burnt match or a weathered Q-tip towering over nearby houses.

Sandor Firenczi, Freud's colleague, "described body parts as having their own 'organ eroticism,'" which Moore understands to mean "that each organ has its own private life and personality that takes pleasure in its activities...that the body's parts not only function...but it takes pleasure in what they do. One asks, not is the organ working, but is it enjoying itself." So—more than one authority blesses my talking to my body...

Paracelsus said, "The physician should speak of that which is invisible. What is visible should belong to his knowledge, and he should recognize illnesses, just as anyone who is not a physician can recognize them from their symptoms. But this is far from making him a physician; he becomes a physician only when he knows that which is unnamed, invisible, and immaterial, yet has its affect." I wonder if modern physicians ever stumble upon that statement in their years of medical education.

...The saw drones on. Now the man in the cherry-picker is paring down the bulbous head that is all that remains of the bushy treetop that greeted this morning's sunrise...

Moore continues, "...all illness is stereophonic. It plays out at the level of actual body tissues and also at the level of the dream. All illness is meaningful....We need to feel the truth of the god within the illness in order to be cured by the disease...we do not cure diseases, they cure us, by restoring our religious participation in life. If the gods appear in our diseases, it follows that our lives may be too secular and in need of such a visitation." For me, RA is the syndrome that is symbolic of all that is unsettled in my body, mind, soul.

...Decapitated now, the pitiful palm is disappearing, and the man in the cherry-picker drones on.

Sunday, February 5, 1995

Rain and I went to San Gregorio beach this morning. I shivered on the sand while she waded barefoot in the surf at the same time Kev was camping in -11° weather in the Porcupine Mountains in upper Michigan!

Living inside for months at a time, it's easy to have a small idea of what life is. Being on the beach, even for half an hour, or being outdoors anywhere, especially at night, reminds me that there are things much greater, much older, much deeper. Earth is a minuscule portion of creation, and humankind even smaller.

Monday, February 20, 1995

Presidents' Day, a holiday from work...Radio and TV news today contained the usual measure of gung-ho drivel about our "near-perfect" system of freedom but I believe that we Americans, and perhaps other first-worlders, are no less enslaved than second- and third-worlders. Whereas they have been physically and politically and economically taken over by empire predators and economic colonialists, we're enslaved by the idea of the inevitability and supremacy of materialism and the amount of time and energy its care and feeding consumes. However, we are relatively physically comfortable in our enslavement, and they are not, and that obviously makes all the difference.

The difference may be temporary, however, because according to Paul Hawken in *The Ecology of Commerce,* "...industrialism itself may not last for even one more lifetime" and anyone can guess which will be the next step in our economic evolution.

Hawken quotes Ivan Illich who pointed out that "...the average American is involved with his or her automobile— working in order to buy it, actually driving it, getting it repaired, and so on—for sixteen hundred hours a year. This means when all car mileage in a given year is divided by the time spent supporting the car, the average car owner is travelling at an average speed of five miles per hour. To attain the speed of a bicycle, we are devastating our cities, lungs, and lives, while bringing on the threat of global warming." I wonder what difference, if any, such realization might have to industrialism and developing countries—or to me.

Tuesday, February 21, 1995

I've been flaring for more than a month now and rushing back and forth from herbs to homeopathy to loving my disease as suggested in John Harrison's book, *Love Your Disease*. Harrison's words remind me that there are sometimes *advantages* to being ill. One of the most obvious advantages for me is that friends are often willing to excuse me from some of the usual social obligations even without my asking; another is that people sometimes assume that I can't do certain things before I've even tried. One of the funniest examples of the willingness of people to help, and of their confusion about what constitutes help, happened in the San Jose airport last summer when I was returning from Michigan.

De-planing at the San Jose airport is done via a roll-up stairway directly onto the tarmac rather than through the familiar tunnel to the terminal used in most airports. Since I can't yet descend stairs in the usual feet-pointed-forward left-right-left way and I must go down sideways, slowly, like a small child, I try to wait until most other passengers have moved past me in the aisle so I won't slow their progress down the stairs. But that's not always possible; sometimes I'm just sort of swept up into the middle of the rushing pack of passengers and we're all stuck with my slower pace once I get to the stairs.

Last summer, as I was side-stepping down the stairs and slowing everyone else down, a well-meaning man behind me grabbed my left elbow, thus lifting that side of me and surprising me almost off balance, then shouted directly into my ear, "DO YA NEED SOME HELP?" His heart was in the right place but his common sense was nowhere around; did he think I was side-stepping because I had a hearing problem?

Harrison writes, "When we have established our investment in creating and maintaining our disease, we can decide to achieve the advantages (and these may include attention, solitude, love, respite from work, and others) in less painful and damaging ways. That is, we can learn to get what we want without needing a disease to justify it." I'm tempted to be incensed, even outraged, at the suggestion that I might be malingering, yet deep down I must acknowledge that RA does have its good points. And I remember a Saturday in April of 1971 when, after seeing a TV ad soliciting donations for the Arthritis Foundation, I thought to myself that, if I ever had a serious or chronic illness, I would want a 'clean' disease, like arthritis, that doesn't (I thought then) involve bleeding or bodily secretion of any kind. Was that some kind of self-fulfilling prophesy?

Do I employ too many outside teachers and influences at once? Maybe. But maybe, with Brooke Medicine Eagle in *White Buffalo Woman Comes Singing,* I might reason that "the Great Spirit needs to give us hard-headed ones several teachers to knock powerfully on the door of our consciousness…I go around and around again, through level after level of learning on a particular issue…I fully expect to be learning until I leave this body."

Maybe the ultimate foolishness is to expect a different result from the same old action—changing my focus almost daily from one philosophy to another, or mixing therapies. Maybe it's time to change that pattern and choose only one philosophy or therapy; but which one?

Thursday, February 23, 1995

My left shoulder has been much better all day although it was stiff when I woke up, and my foot spurs were large and painful. My right foot was swollen in the afternoon. My right shoulder and both hips were painful most of the day and my neck and jaw have been stiff. My right foot was swollen and spongy, especially above my great toe, all evening.

The mercurial nature of this disease is so exasperating. Symptoms change from hour to hour but now I wonder if my

RA is actually receding and it is *osteoarthritis,* which my allopathic physician diagnosed as a minor component of my illness, that is causing my current problems. I can't recall when I last had a hot joint and now, even when I do have joint inflammation, it's relatively slight and brief. On the other hand, the problems I have now seem to be more the result of inadequate tendons and cartilage which are features of both types of arthritis. To test this idea I'm going to try a combination of glucosamine sulfate (for the osteoarthritic component of my problem), tissue salts, flax oil, anti-oxidants and herbs.

Friday, February 24, 1995

My shoulders, back, and neck were much better during the night but crunchy and more painful when I got up. The hunching in my shoulders has finally let down. I was able to raise both arms above my head, while lying down, for the first time in awhile. My knees are sore but my hips feel fine. My toes are bunching, my wrists are sore.

Monday, February 27, 1995

My left shoulder is a lot better; everything else is a little better.

"Every word, thought or uttered, has some effect," Connie Fillmore writes in *The Unity Guide To Healing,* "Every word brings forth after its kind…Words of weakness change to weakness the character of everything that receives them. Talking…will produce corresponding conditions in the body; on the other hand, sending forth the word of strength and affirming power will bring about strength and poise." In other words, if I think I must take a remedy, or fast, to regain my health, it thereby becomes a fact; or if I affirm I am well or ill, it becomes so. Is this true? Many writers I respect think so.

I seem no longer to have active RA although I certainly do still have the scars and deformity from having had it in the past. I don't know about other diseases, or others' diseases, but I know that somehow my dis-ease—from RA to OA to depression to spiritual anguish to guilt and feelings of inadequacy—have been based on or caused by *fear.*

Fear about my ability to earn a living has set up an endless loop of circular reality; *fear* about my ability to be well enough to earn a living causes my RA to flare which makes, in fact, my ability to earn a living more dubious and escalates the original fear. And *fear* about my general adequacy, my inability to accept common wisdom about the purposes of life and the way to live, and even *fear* of life itself cause me to lose all perspective, to lose my *self* in trying to fit in or measure up or defend against. Yet I imagine that, if I were to carefully and consistently follow my own lights, reinforced by the most believable others I can find, my health problems would dissolve, or at least recede further.

All my most respectable teachers express the idea in quite similar phrasing that what takes place physically has first taken place in some mind. I *know* that I have created my dis-ease. Of course I haven't done so by directly declaring my intention to have rheumatoid arthritis or osteoarthritis, to be depressed or discontent. I've done so by painting a picture in my mind of what I *don't* want, rather than what I *do* want, and by a mechanism I can't explain but I know is fact—somehow—my sub-conscious, or the universe, or God, or nature, or whomever or whatever, using roving opportunistic pathogens, fulfills that picture. I'm not sure of many things but of this one idea I'm as certain as I can be of anything; but I easily lose my grip on this idea, or simply lose track of it when I'm doing well.

The reason I lose faith is that I am too easily influenced by the world around me which usually doesn't even acknowledge that such a concept exists much less that it has validity. And I *fear*—*fear,* again—that this concept is just too easy, representative only of my wish, coincidental, that its manifestations are my misinterpretations of events and truth.

When I regain myself and calmly contemplate my life and my own lights and understanding and intuitions, my fears dissipate. When I become grandiose in my planning, when I live too much in the future or in the past, when I try to fit in or fit a role, my disease flares in the form of RA, OA, depression, digestive distress, etc.

If I must be swayed by others, let it be by those who *speculate* rather than those who are *certain* that they have captured truth. Let it be from among those who wonder whether life is a school or a workshop or a play—in which we all choose our own costumes and roles and lines, as we go along, or even before birth…

Friday, March 3, 1995

I was feeling worse when I woke up; was it the lentil soup, sesame pasta, and bagel I ate yesterday? I've taken *rhus tox,* aspirin, and cold and hot compresses and, now, an hour later, the pain is subsiding. I remember that prior to 1992 it was necessary for me to get up more than two hours earlier than I needed to in order to get ready for the day and for work, to allow time for my stiff body to limber up and for the morning dose of aspirin to kill enough pain for me to move around.

I wonder if I have confused my case by using more than one therapy at a time; because of that possibility I'm thinking of starting over with another fast but I'm conflicted about that too. To what extent does my faith invest anything—therapy, food, fast, spiritual exercise—with the power to change my health or my life? Am I addressing the root of my problem with material changes alone? Would spiritual means alone be adequate?

Maybe the answer to that question is "yes." According to Corinne McLaughlin and Gordon Davidson in *Spiritual Politics,* "A number of studies have all demonstrated the capacity of the immune system to respond to intentional behavioral strategies and mental visualization." And according to Andrew Weil, in *The Natural Mind,* "The only limits we encounter in the world around us are those we first create in our imagination." In *The Aquarian Conspiracy,* Marilyn Ferguson concludes, "What our self-identity is will determine how we will recreate our biology and our environment." All of these statements seem to me more true than statements to the contrary by other researchers; on the other hand, I want to believe that matter is controlled by spirit rather than the other way around.

Ferguson writes,

> Everything of importance is already known, a sage said—
> the only thing is to rediscover it. Much of the current
> excitement about healing is a kind of collective
> remembering and homecoming to the old wives and
> old doctors. Hippocrates, with his insistence on the
> importance of mind and milieu could have warned us of
> the consequences of medical pigeonholing....Like the foil
> wrap on a disappointing gift, the shiny technology has dealt
> stunningly with certain acute problems...but its failure in
> chronic and degenerative disease...have driven practitioners
> and patients to look elsewhere...holistic health originates in

an attitude; an acceptance of life's uncertainties, a willingness to accept responsibility for habits, a way of perceiving and dealing with stress, more satisfying human relationships, a sense of purpose.

Saturday, March 11, 1995 — 1 p.m.

For the past twelve days I've been taking flax caps and anti-oxidant tabs daily; the result has been a slight reduction in pain, especially at night. When I started this regime, night pain and stiffness had been escalating. My shoulders, wrists, and knees had been very bad every morning. Since I've been on the regime my toes, feet, hips, fingers, elbows, clavicle, neck had been less painful while my ribs and jaw are slightly improved. I decided at about eleven this morning to discontinue the medications and to begin the fast I'd been planning to start next Wednesday.

7:10 p.m.

My foot spurs are pretty bad and my toes are bunching. Twinges in left wrist and right knee are bothersome. My hands are stiff and painful. Both shoulders are stiff and painful when I try to raise my arms.

I'm planning to go in to work as usual on Monday and Tuesday; I wonder how that will be.

10 p.m.

I'm neither weak nor cold, as some books I've read suggest I might be, but am I hungry! I've had about seventy-two ounces of fluids today, a little more than most authorities recommend. I think I'm not drinking for thirst but for hunger. My eyes seem unusually dry.

Sunday, March 12, 1995 — 8:30 a.m.

Pain and stiffness were bad enough when I first got up this
morning but not nearly as bad as three years ago when I
started my first fast. I'm hungry but my stomach is not
grumbling and uncomfortable like yesterday. Now that
I've been up for about half an hour, pain and stiffness have
diminished somewhat, even without aspirin, food, or drink.

9 a.m.

Alfalfa tea tastes, feels, smells wonderful!

According to my reading, autolysis, which will result in
the breakdown of all my spurs and nodules and plates, begins
approximately on day four; that would be Tuesday. If I break
my fast on Friday, I'll have had three days of autolysis. Should
I try to wait until Saturday to break my fast?

I'm feeling anxious and irritated that I have chores to do
today and that I'm committed to working tomorrow and
Tuesday—also that enemas are necessary during fasting and
that I must take one this morning.

Unless I keep moving, my wrists are stiff and painful. I'm
warm but I'm not perspiring. I feel better, I think, when I'm
perspiring.

A sunny morning; the street is quiet; a few cars pass; a
BART train whistles. I watched a few minutes of TV news
yesterday and a half-hour of stand-up comedy but, otherwise,
I've minimized my intake of everything. I sat outside for
awhile trying to just be there without mental activity but
didn't succeed. Stilling my mind in any type of meditation is
difficult; I'm so undisciplined. Fortunately, according to
Raymond Van Over and Alan Watts, both meditation experts,
even the occasional unsuccessful effort can be restorative. I've
been convinced about the marvels of meditation for a long

time but I spend more time reading and talking and writing *about* it that *practicing* it.

11 a.m.

Is it my imagination, or wishful thinking, or are the whites of my eyes more clear, my face pinker, healthier-looking? I'm feeling not exactly weak but a pleasant, calm heaviness.

12:30 p.m.

Listened to Beethoven's *Symphony No. 9 in D Minor*—just right for the occasion.

I've had no aspirin for about thirty-six hours and I'm not feeling much pain at all. My knees are snapping a bit and my hands and wrists hurt a little. My feet are sore, the spurs are sharp. I have the same backache I occasionally have at work.

I'm a little sore, a little slow, a little heavy, but I'm sure I can easily work and safely drive. It's more than forty-eight hours since I've eaten and I would like to eat—but I'm not ravenous.

Monday, March 13, 1995 — 7:15 a.m.

It's very warm in my room which is good for my joints but my mouth, nose, eyes are all dry. I'm stiff. My wrists are painful. My hands are a shaky—is autolysis beginning or do I tremble due to low blood sugar? I wish I hadn't planned to work today. Sixty hours since I've had food, almost at the halfway point. Forty-eight hours since I've had aspirin. Is it my imagination or is the nodule in my right elbow smaller?

4:15 p.m.

I was feeling tired, weak, shaky at work so I left early. It's odd not to have food planning, prep, clean-up and eating to punctuate the day. Eating is a very pleasurable activity for me; I live to eat as much as I eat to live, I guess.

Tuesday, March 14, 1995 — 7:30 a.m.

I'm hot, weak, shaky. My knees are stinging; my wrists are sore. My toes are bunching together and the spurs stab as I walk. My upper arms are banding and stinging. The top of my right foot is sore as are the tendons in my neck. My shoulders are fairly comfortable. I've had no aspirin for three days but I can tolerate this level of pain without it. Autolysis should be in process. I wish I hadn't committed to working today; I am looking forward to five days of retreat, of concentrating on physical and spiritual cleansing and renewal.

The neighbor's gardener was working earlier with his fume-spewing leaf-blower and the exhaust stench hangs heavily over the neighborhood. Raindrops fall softly beyond the overhang but only a few sift down through the oak.

I've decided not to do enemas any more—they seem too unnatural. Other animals, whose example I often find helpful, do fast when they're not feeling well but they don't do enemas.

Wednesday, March 15, 1995 — 7:30 a.m.

When I awoke, everything was comfortable—not perfectly so, but much better—especially my wrists and shoulders and neck. My right knee is a bit tender. My foot spurs are smaller—but sharper!

I'm in my fifth day of abstaining from food and aspirin. I'm looking for excuses to begin breaking my fast as soon as possible although I notice that I feel better without the fruit juices and vegetable broth I've been taking, when I'm taking only tea and water. All of the juices are now too sweet.

It appears to be true that Christian Scientists, for example, can somehow avoid addressing the material aspects of healing and curing but I think I cannot—not right now at any rate. I think that this fast is the next phase of my healing. The autolytic process is cleansing my body of unwanted and unneeded tissue—diseased tissue, toxins, abscesses, cysts, tumors, fat deposits, mineral deposits, lumps, nodules, overgrowths, anything that doesn't belong where it is, in order to permit healthy, easy function and regeneration of healthy new tissue. Fasting erases the effects of my bad habits and eliminates temporary allergies and food sensitivities that have developed so I can start over, eating virtually anything in prudent quantities and patterns and combinations.

When I resume eating, will it be better to endure, and be thus preoccupied with, the inconvenience and self-denial of never again eating an unhealthy thing? Is it better to suffer with the pain and physical limitation resulting from, and preoccupation with, longer-term ill effects of eating whatever I wish? Perhaps a mixture of the two by usually eating wisely and only occasionally eating poorly and trusting that my body will be able to withstand the occasional lapses? I'm so sick of being ruled by health considerations, of always being focussed on ill health!

I'm making yellow pea soup for Rain. An article I read recently suggested that merely smelling food provides some appetite satisfaction. Let's see…

Friday, March 17, 1995

Reborn strawberry plants with a few ambitious blossoms, under the tangerine tree, reinforce the idea that regeneration and recovery are also facts of life. The rotting tangerine I squashed underfoot adds its alcoholic perfume to the bouquet of moist earth and damp pine needles. Some heavier scent wafts in and out—is it freesia? The sky is so blue, the clouds so white, the leaves so glossy and clean. Is it star jasmine?

Consider how far I have come in the last three years. Cortisone enabled me to visit California. Fasting and homeopathy enabled me to visit Madison, to move to California, to visit Portland and Tulsa and Tacoma. Homeopathy, herbs, acupuncture, and better nutrition enabled me to become stronger, then to start walking. Walking has enabled me to grow even stronger and to walk even farther. The more I've done, the more I've been able to do.

Saturday, March 18, 1995

I broke my fast today. My joints are much better but my spurs are not. I wonder whether I should have fasted longer. I'm also suspicious of the fruit juice I was drinking. Should I have done a water-only fast?

Saturday, March 25, 1995

I'm feeling so well but I'm not back to normal eating yet. Rain and I had a very *careful* lunch together and went to a matinee showing of *Before the Rain*. It's been a lovely warm day and there's still a bit of sunshine left and I don't want to leave it alone outside.

Sunday, May 14, 1995 — Mothers' Day

Rain and I spent yesterday afternoon together at the powwow.
It rained most of that time so we got drenched while sitting
in the bleachers during grand entry. Our shoes and the legs of
our pants were soon mud-dappled as later we worked our way
among the traders' booths. There seemed to be fewer traders
than usual but that may have been mostly due to the forecast
of rain. Of course we ate vegetarian blue corn Indian tacos,
fry bread, and wojapi.

Wednesday, August 9, 1995 — 4 a.m.

It's impossible to sleep with the windows open and too hot
to close them so I've abandoned the hope of sleeping. Kev's
street, State Street in Madison, Wisconsin, still teems with
mourners of the death of Jerry Garcia of the Grateful Dead; it's
been like a flashback to the sixties. State Street is a pedestrian
mall so people, mostly students at the University here, mill
around, beating drums off and on, and talk, now loudly, now
softly. Sometimes I hear a radio.

The police are doing nothing to break up this peaceful
crowd of teens and twenty-somethings who seem stunned by
the passing of this icon of many of their parents. I'm amazed
that so many young people have noticed and cared.

Friday, August 11, 1995

I'm sitting on the lawn at the Roadstar Motel in Madison,
trying to dry my hair in 80% relative humidity and trying to
avoid the chlorine-laden refrigerated air inside. Across the
highway the land rolls easily into farm country; its sky seems
so big, so wide, because buildings and trees are far off. Without
a breeze the still air is heavy and hard to suck into the nostrils,
harder still to drag down into lungs. It's still very hot; a heat

index of a 110° was predicted for today—I wonder if it got
that hot.

Finally a little breeze kicks up. These are the breezes of my
youth—moist, hot, laden with frying fish…

Shy pink sunset, its act aborted
does an embarrassed curtain call after
a hot hard shower,
smells fish fry,
watches traffic resume
in the doorway of the hardware
selling peat and play sand
by the bushel.

The hay-scented breeze which has made my eyes heavy
with sleep—but not parched like my dried-out California
eyes—is large, one-piece, like a bedsheet. In the Bay area, the
breezes are break-away strands from an unravelling ball of
wind. In Wisconsin the wind sticks together; in California
each breeze individuates, does its own thing, and moves on.

Now I sit on the edge of my Roadstar Queen, facing a
full-length mirror that disabuses me once again of any notion
that my body, which has been in my service for fifty-seven
years now, is more shapely, less pasty than those of my peers.
I am bandy of leg and bony of shoulder, this mirror reveals,
and much of my substance has settled as far south as it can
reach while I'm seated. Seated, my base is very solid, like a
Weeble; standing, I look much less stable on my skinny
legs, topographical maps of my circulatory system coursing,
meandering like Indian mounds up and down my beigeness.
Twenty-five years of rheumatoid arthritis have gnarled my
knees and feet like cypress on a windward hillside, or old rose

roots. This inn-keeper must have a particularly cruel streak to install so many full-length mirrors in such unavoidable spots.

Monday, August 14, 1995

Now I'm back home in East Detroit—oops! East Pointe— Michigan. This little city which was called Halfway when my dad was born here in 1916, and later became East Detroit, has recently changed its name again. Variety is the spice of life, I guess.

Back among my brothers and sister, it's as if I saw them all yesterday and we're children again, even though they're getting gray like me, or bald. We joke that we're orphans now that Mom and Dad are both gone—but maybe they're not gone since they're still a main topic of conversation.

It's pretty hard to be a vegan in these parts; although this Detroit metropolitan area is *car* country—or the rust belt, depending upon who's doing the labeling—farmer breakfasts reign! Eggs, bacon or sausage or ham, and hashed brown potatoes are the basics to which toast, pancakes, waffles, grits, and cereal may be added. A vegetarian lunch means a salad of iceberg lettuce—period. But I'm trying to revisit my Michigan life so I eat, with gusto, the greasy hamburger with fried onions, the farmer breakfast with a double order of bacon, extra crisp, thanks, and the White Castle sliders and Buscemi subs.

I spend an afternoon digging through the Burton Collection at the Detroit Main Library, looking for clues to the public lives of our ancestors, then days locating tombstones. I had decades to do these things while I lived here; they seem urgent now that the opportunity comes only annually. At the family picnic, I spend hours listening to Auntie Vi, not an aunt

at all but my dad's first cousin, and the oldest living member of
my dad's family, whose prodigious memory holds all the begats
since the early twenties. She remembers my birth date as well
as those of the other three cousins born in 1938. I visit Aunt
Millie, the only living member of my mom's ten siblings. The
weather is hot and humid, there's no rain in sight, but I'm
drenched in family.

I spend afternoons driving around looking at the sites
of my life. Sacred Heart School, where I attended Saturday
morning catechism classes until I was in grade four, had rented
the high school building to a Baptist academy the last time
I looked, and now the building is gone and the land is an
extension of the old cemetery, which had been full for years,
where some of our relatives lie in their eternal rest.

St. Veronica School, which I attended for grades four
through eight, looks the same although I know it's staffed now
by only a few nuns and many lay teachers because the Sisters
of St. Joseph are dwindling—not enough new vocations, I
guess. I must visit sometime when the school is not locked up
tight for summer to see whether the ghosts of Sr. Euphemia,
Sr. Ambrosia, Sr. Priscilla, Sr. Anita, and Mrs. Verville haunt
those dry halls.

The old wooden St. Gertrude church, built before the
turn of the century, if I recall correctly, has been replaced by
something modern and nondescript and too close to the road.
That high school building—my high school for two years—
has also been rented to a fundamentalist church group; my
heart floods with bitter and sweet memories—Sr. Agnella,
who suggested I might think about writing; my first boyfriend,
the bass drummer; roller-skating parties; Rene's grocery store
where, when I had baby-sitting money, I would buy a one-
pound bag of Hekman's chocolate drop cookies and eat the
entire contents while waiting for our chartered Greyhound
bus. The grade-school building is still there; if I were to climb

the three long flights of stairs to the band's attic practice room, would I find "my" cello waiting in its stand for me to try again to correctly count the thirty-two measures of its "In a Persian Marketplace" solo? Across the street, Lake St. Clair, on which we skated during winter lunch hours, in which we swam at every opportunity, is as blue as ever.

I drive past Lucy's childhood house, now occupied by strangers, then visit her mom in a nursing home; she's in her late eighties and doesn't remember me although Lucy and I were inseparable from fourth grade through our marriages. In 1954 she taught me to say *"¿A tenido usted un buen día?"* which I've never forgotten, but she, alas, in her sweet Spanish old age, has forgotten me. I'm glad I visited her nonetheless.

I revisit Bishop Lake where we had so many family picnics, where my brothers the Boy Scouts camped so many summers, where we nearly incinerated ourselves one March rushing the picnic season and trying to cook hot dogs while wearing mittens. Ah, memories…

Saturday, September 2, 1995

Why do I watch the news? There's never anything new; it seems that most varieties of human experience are going on at all times. There's always a greater war and lesser wars, prosperity and poverty, great strength and great weakness, inspired leaders and charlatans of every stripe, natural disasters, human excesses and deficiencies, people seeking answers to ponderous questions and those who think they have all the answers, those who wouldn't presume to teach and those who would impose their enlightenment by any means necessary.

Maybe I watch the news for the same reason I read—to find clues to the mystery of what I'm supposed to do in this life. Are we meant to merely exist for awhile and follow urges?

Every day I vacillate yet, often enough, the fog seems to clear and I'm convinced we've been placed here by a force outside ourselves for its unrevealed purposes.

I'm glad that I can believe in a greater, however unfathomable to me and indescribable by me, Intelligence which/who has caused all of what I can know, my ability to know, and all that there is to know. I'm glad that I can often enough trust that "Out of Grace I cannot fall," that all will work out in the end and that the end is somehow beyond this current conscious experience.

I'm glad that the way I seem to be at my best is evidence to me that God is great, God is good, as some children are taught to say in blessing food before they eat, and that there must be some spiritual heaven, beyond bodily death, of which the good aspects of this life are a foreshadowing. Yet I doubt there is a hell beyond, of which the hellish aspects of this life are a foreshadowing.

But why would I assume that the larger life is happy when it's obvious that I have both good and evil inclinations (evil being destructive or anti-social acts)? Why would I not reason that the mix would continue into the larger life, that gods war as we humans do? I don't understand my inconsistencies along these lines but, for the moment at least, I can live with them. How do I know there must finally be one "god"? My brain, my capacity to understand, cannot venture so far, can explain no more.

Am I living as I should; is there a blueprint anywhere? As near as I can tell, every life and all its parts are original works of art—even the healing component—although healing can't be the basis of a life. Healing oneself can only be part of the *housekeeping* of a life; living healthily, healing, replaces living unhealthily, illness. The process is not to erase illness and then, later, color in health but more like healthy acts being wedged into an unhealthy life and displacing unhealthy practices in the process. But wherever an individual is on the wellness/illness scale can only be part of the *context* of living, not its purpose.

Afternoon westerlies play for gay green leaves
who dance and sway in clean September air
and shame me from my pondering the same weighty matters
I pondered in January's winds and November's damp
and many an earlier September's breezes,
and bid me relax today contemplating
what to be known must be felt.

Tuesday, September 5, 1995 — evening

Summer seems to be as Indian as it gets here on the peninsula. For two or three days now, the hot hot daytime air has seemed almost Michigan fresh. The sky is—well—sky blue during the bright days and bright night blue after dark as a great number of stars come out to take the balmy evening air. Kinfolk of the hordes of sweat bees I fought for my bratwurst in Madison a mere month ago, engage me in battle yet again—this time for my chocolate biscotti; none bother to threaten or to sting, they simply want food, you hear? Food!

Life is good! The children are well and happy and living in places a mother feels no call to fudge about and both have nice friends. The relatives are all speaking to each other and I had a wonderful shopping excursion.

I found a wonderful pair of well-tailored, all-cotton, made-in-the-USA pants, in a great color, for a fair price, at a nearby store and, wonder of wonders, they fit! Standing, the seat neither clings nor sags; seated, the fabric pulls not across the thigh. Guaranteed never to need ironing, soft but not flimsy, with a sturdy zipper, an un-ugly waistband button, un-thready belt loops, these pants are my new favorite garment that I'll love for a long time. But, alas, there's just the teeniest, tiniest, wispiest fly in this wonderful ointment—not much, but just enough to take the edge off my ecstacy; I probably shouldn't think of it at all. After all, perfection exists nowhere in this vale of tears so I won't even mention it—but I just can't get it out of my mind. I got them in the men's department.

Tuesday, September 12, 1995

The morning fog creates an interval between night and day, suitable for stock-taking and planning. The appearance of the sun at eleven or so is the signal for the day to begin.

My knees grind as I rise to fetch pistachios for Markus N. Backus, our resident black squirrel with the z-shaped mark on his back. He has already devoured the corn chip I left perched on a little wart on the trunk of the oak. He takes his three pistachios, one by one, from their place on top of my shod foot and devours them, then walks round and round my chair, rising on hind legs every few inches to look me squarely in the eye as if to say "Well???"
Eventually he starts to climb the leg of my chair but I'm afraid he'll use those tough little jaws, which can make such short shrift of unopenable pistachios, to bite me so I fetch a length of pretzel which he carries high up into the tree to eat. I hear him munching.

In my mind, this illness, and certainly this last small portion of which I'm still trying to heal, has never been permanent even though it's over twenty-five years old; I've always considered it a temporary condition. The reason it's lasted until now is that for so long I used the wrong therapies and my belief in them was never strong enough for them to work as placebos.

What has happened in my body? My connective tissue has been weak so my various organs, tissues, bones, systems, are no longer in proper alignment and relationship to each other. Parts of my body have shifted and distorted when stressed and not all have returned to their proper places; misalignment has bred misalignment. Sometimes to compensate, or in the confusion of being overwhelmed, my body still produces plates and nodes and nodules and spurs of excess materials too heavy to circulate and deposits them in places like my soles, the tops of my feet, as bands around my upper arm bones, in my finger and toe and shoulder joints.

My feet and ankles have slipped out of proper alignment as I have walked on my flattened arches and my tendons have been too weak to pull everything back into proper place. My arms, shoulders, and neck have been pulled out of proper relationship by the weight of my arms, by my sleeping positions, etc., and my ligaments and tendons have been too weak to restore them.

The underlying cause of all this is weak, unhealthy, inadequate collagen, the material that gives strength and integrity to connective tissue. Could the reason my connective tissue is weak be that it is expressing my deep belief and *fear* that I can't hold *myself* and my life together?

I still believe my illness is temporary, if long, like the boy in *How Green Was My Valley;* as miraculously as he healed, I am healing, I believe. Medical science says my deformity itself cannot be healed but I think it can.

I know I somehow unconsciously chose and capitulated to this disease sometime around 1970 as a defense against impossible stresses. I also know that physical manifestations are the easiest to change while the underlying psychological or survival problems are harder to solve, but still solvable. Our bodies are equipped for self-healing—not just of simple ailments or other people's ailments—but of RA and all ailments, I'm convinced.

Sunday, September 17, 1995

I'm relearning how it feels to toss a sheet or blanket over the far edge of the bed, rather than to laboriously walk each corner around; each day I do it more easily and comfortably. It's been a long time since I've made these movements.

Rain will soon be here for breakfast and to connect my new printer for me and hang my new Monet print. I can't quite do such things yet but there's no hurry, no need for anxiety about time. My dearest, oldest friend Lucy, who died too soon, in 1987, can still be a model for me of healthy attitudes toward time and patience.

The more I concentrate on fear and worry, the more I harm my body. Negative expectations make me sick. My unconscious mind makes me sick and my unconscious mind makes me well. My unconscious mind directs my body to make real what my conscious mind pictures.

Tuesday, October 3, 1995

I still have my veil fetish, I realize as I watch Benazir Bhutto on TV. She looks like a modern-day madonna in her silky white veil draping so gracefully over her glossy black hair and framing her aristocratic face. Serenely she waits, while interviewer Charlie Rose slogs through rambling questions, then articulates a concise response. Her grace and physical beauty accentuate her obvious intelligence. She's a credit to her veil.

Lidian Emerson, the wife of Ralph Waldo Emerson, appearing demure, modest, and chaste, graces a chin-length veil resting lightly on shining hair in a nineteenth-century photograph. Dark-skinned women in many parts of the world, sheets of long dark hair, living veils swinging in elegant counterpoint to un-self-conscious rhythms of sturdy bodies, step bare-footed through their days. Sometimes they carry burdens, like heavy crowns, on their heads. They do their veils honor.

I fell in love with the idea of being a nun at one 6:30 a.m. Sunday mass when I was entranced by the veils of the Sisters of St. Joseph.

As altar boys folded the white communion cloth, section by section, over the marble communion rail, the Sisters would slip beaded pins from their moorings to allow the fold-back of their sheer black, waist-length veils to fall forward to cover the starched white bands that stood, crown-like, above downcast eyes.

Then they'd remove more pins to un-cuff voluminous black outer sleeves to allow them to fall gracefully over fitted black inner sleeves and cover all but the tips of their fingers. The whole row of black serge and black veiling would sway out of the first pew on St. Joseph's altar side and glide silently to the communion rail to receive holy communion, the trans-substantiated body and blood of Christ, to be followed by the other St. Veronica Church parishioners.

Palms flattened against each other, pointing heavenward, holding those sleeves in place, like garments to be grown into, the sisters would float back to their pew. By the time the rest of us had returned from the rail and had spent the appropriate five minutes praying silently with our hands covering our faces, the Sisters would have refolded their veils and sleeves and would be kneeling motionless, faceless cones of black as the altar boys restored the communion cloth to its original position. Veils called me to the convent.

Saturday, October 28, 1995

Another sweet October afternoon. I'm torn between reading and writing outside and doing accounting work inside.— Okay, I'll do the accounting later, after dark which comes too early these days, and not miss being out in so perfect a day. On such a day, how is it possible that the greatest portion of the world is cold, starving, exploited, oppressed, abused, and/or at war when I am warm, dry, fed, loved, and relatively safe?

I hear "Johnny Be Good" played by a band in Mitchell Park and see five tiny lemon-winged butterflies flitting among the late coral rose-buds. A warm breeze passes over my bare arms. I have laryngitis.

My beloved daughter calls to discuss the relative merits of wool-fill and cotton-fill in the comforter she plans to buy but urges me not to challenge my laryngitic vocal cords by whispering. We spent a lovely time together yesterday evening, visiting a new book shop, sharing a Chinese dinner, and viewing *A Scent Of Green Papaya* on video at her place. Like old times in Wixom, we shared an Almond Joy, a Bit o' Honey, and Reese's Peanut Butter Cups. I'm so lucky.

In *Mother Jones* magazine I read an interview of Gloria Steinem at 61, in which she observes that many women as they age become more radical whereas, as men age, they tend to become more conservative. I'd like to find some way, radical or otherwise, that would help heal all the wounded things around us, but what I find is small ways that sometimes make small inroads.

Are all the things that I see as evil—greed, arrogance, and power lust—elemental evil, or are they the result of ignorance and/or fear? Are they perhaps the result of too little thought and a way of reasoning that, since a first response to a problem seems reasonable and inevitable, all other responses must be wrong?

I wish I had a strong *conviction* that we live many earthly incarnations; it would be such a consolation. If I were sure of what I should do, however small, I would feel better. Contributing money just can't be enough.

I want to remember more often that, although I can't directly change much, I can, by the butterfly effect, indirectly and subtly change everything. I want to more fully observe Buddhist principles of right living and right livelihood, Jesus' command to love one another, Quaker principles of listening for the voice of God, Emerson's advice on the conduct of life: to escape all false ties, to have the courage to be what I am, to love what is simple and beautiful, to live independently but in cheerful relation to all else, to serve, to add somewhat to the general well-being.

Thursday, November 2, 1995

It's definitely fall and I've been feeling like digging myself in for the winter since daylight saving time ended yet I miss working outside for long periods. Even here in the sun I'm cool.

I wish everyone in the world had at least at much as I have; then I'd feel comfortable thinking mostly of myself.

Thursday, December 23, 1995

Solstice yesterday at San Gregorio Beach was quiet, solemn. The beach was smooth and clear since the usual scattered debris had been pushed hard into a black tangle against the cliffs by the last weeks' storms.

No birds were on the beach and none were playing in the surf although a few black birds with yellow eyes meandered, like migrating cells, among the black debris and other birds soared and wheeled overhead in the watery air and sculptured sunbeams.

Only a few other people were there, far fewer than on Thanksgiving Wednesday when Rain and Brad and I inspected a few of the shallow caves carved into the cliffs by the water, when the fog was so heavy that only a few yards of surf were visible from the sand. We walked the beach for about an hour, picking up trash, then left, drenched, to dry out by the car heater. Later we went to see *Carrington.*

It's cold but I'm writing outside because I have recently read a couple of books on the subject of natural light as nutrient and as therapy. James Winston Benfield, D.D.S., in his introduction to John N. Ott's book, *Health and Light,* writes, "Research has now demonstrated that the full spectrum of daylight is important to stimulate man's endocrine system properly and that he suffers side effects when forced to spend much of his time under artificial light sources that reproduce only a limited portion of the daylight spectrum." Now I suspect that it's lack of sunlight that has started me into an arthritic flare, toward the end of each of the years I've been here, and kept the flares going each time until late spring when I would finally, in desperation, begin another course of professional treatment. In Ott's book he tells the story of how his crippling RA dramatically improved after circumstances kept him outdoors in natural light without reading glasses or sunglasses and of his subsequent research in the area of light; it's a fascinating book.

Jacob Liberman in *Light: Medicine of the Future* writes,

> The same blue light found to be successful in the
> treatment of neonatal jaundice also has been very effective
> in reducing pain in people with rheumatoid arthritis.
> In 1982, Dr. Sharon McDonald conducted a study on
> 60 middle-aged women with rheumatoid arthritis at the
> San Diego State University School of Nursing.
>
> The purpose of the study was to determine the
> relationship between the degree of pain people experienced
> and the presence of specific visible wave-lengths of light in
> their environments. Utilizing a simply constructed box
> with an ordinary incandescent light source shining through
> a blue filter, Dr. McDonald instructed her subjects to slip
> their hands into the box through a specifically designed
> opening while she shined blue light on their hands for
> varying amounts of time up to fifteen minutes. Although
> this exposure time was short, a significant degree of pain
> relief was experienced by most subjects.

According to Liberman, there are tremendous health
benefits from ultraviolet light. He writes that,

> UV light activates the synthesis of vitamin D, which is
> a prerequisite for the absorption of calcium and other
> minerals from the diet...lowers blood pressure...increases
> the efficiency of the heart...improves electrocardiogram
> (EKG) readings and blood profiles of individuals with
> atherosclerosis (hardening of the arteries)...reduces
> cholesterol...assists in weight loss...is an effective treatment
> for psoriasis...is an effective treatment for many other
> diseases...increases the level of sex hormones...activates an
> important skin hormone.

Wow, that's a lot to hope for from spending time in full-
spectrum light!

So—I'm planning to be outdoors at least an hour each day, in natural light if not in direct sunlight. I may also get a full-spectrum lamp or a light-box to use on the days when it rains or when I can't manage to find an hour to spend outdoors.

Wednesday, December 27, 1995

A glorious day! Unbroken blue sky spreads over leftover holy day quiet. A raven squawks overhead then squats heavily in the orange tree. Vague scent of fresh wood smoke wanders through the still air. Damn! The neighbor's gardener has just arrived and is clanking his mowers and blowers off his truck. Soon we'll be inundated by their roar and the stench of burning fossil fuel—there oughta be a law!

I'm flaring a bit and so are Kev and Rain. My neck has been bothering me for days. My knees are sore and grinding. My upper arms were aching a few minutes ago but now they're fine. The spurs on my soles have been especially painful. Can all this be due to the way I've been eating since Thanksgiving? To lack of sunlight? Am I like the damaged fuchsias suspended from the overhang—too damaged and deformed to be able to return to health, yet able to continue living with the deformity?

…I had to come inside because the neighbor is doing something that is producing a hiss and banana oil smell that was choking me…

Thursday, December 28, 1995

If depression is anger turned inward, then RA is fear turned inward. Every day I realize more that a person governed by fear must *learn* to be bold, brave, and courageous, and must invent, create, imagine, the courage to confront her dragons. I realize that she must at last discover for herself that most dragons are toothless, but that it is better to be *slain* in combat with a dragon than to live, begging for mercy, flashing the soft pink underbelly of RA or any other offspring of fear.

The dilemma is how to confront the dragon. Allopathy does battle by throwing rocks, by tossing broken glass, by using noxious chemicals, by knife attacks, but ends up harming only the victim because the dragon RA is itself an illusion, an effect, a syndrome, a miasma, a figment of who knows whom or what. Naturopathy defends by fortifying with food and supplements. Homeopathy stimulates by mimicking the disease process. Acupuncture prods and goads into health. Religion often blames original and/or subsequent sin and posits a sado-masochistic god, while psychology sometimes blames the victim.

The problem, the dragon RA, may itself be a primeval biological *therapy* preceding schools of medicine/pathology. Or it may be at least partly a symbolic response to avoid battle and being devoured—some diseases will control the honorable dragons outside by shaming them out of doing battle with an unworthy opponent. Interior dragons are controlled by being too weak to address them. It's a way of choosing death by weakness rather than chancing sudden death in battle. RA has prolonged my life by wounding me early so I might be excused from battle—and, unfortunately, from a division of the spoils as well.

I do know that some things are undeniably, universally, physically, materially true: arsenic in lethal amounts will kill, I will quickly die without adequate oxygen. All diseases do have physical manifestations and some have specific pathogens but cause/effect relationship in some diseases are not inevitable or universal or undeniable. The presence of the pathogen does not always indicate or herald the presence of the disease nor does the presence of a syndrome of symptoms necessarily indicate the existence of a physical pathogen, even an undetectable one. There is, after all, a finite number of symptom combinations within the human body/mind so all pathogens, dis-eases, disorders must choose among these and overlap is inevitable.

Tuesday, January 2, 1996

*These things are not optional
our learning and love
must pass
into the genetic coding of the universe.*

Another sunny morning, almost balmy. Smells like the first day of school and the little grove that separated Cliff Read's Funeral Home's parking lot from its neighbors' yards on Toepfer Street on lunch hours, when I would leave the St. Veronica School playground without permission to walk the four blocks to Grandma Hooper's house.

I was always tempted to walk into that tiny forest to pick the tender lilies-of-the-valley whose perfume I could smell from the sidewalk, and the bold pink phlox, strident among the scruffy evergreen and boxwood; I never did, though. As much as I longed to probe that mysterious place, and as much as I wanted those flowers, I feared more that I might find among them a mislaid corpse from the funeral home or maybe evidence of murder and torture, a werewolf, or even a zombie—one of the dreaded un-dead. I would walk nonchalantly past the grove, sniffing greedily, then run as fast as I could the rest of the way to Grandma's or back to school!

Saturday, January 6, 1996

Another glorious California morning without a cloud—
except the ones in my mind. The more comfortable I get, the
more aware and uneasy I become about how lucky I am to be
comfortable while most of the world's populations are under
some sort of siege and barely existing with none or few of
the comforts of either rural life or urban life. In addition to
being—as we lucky few are—only at the mercy of wind and
weather, pestilence and ignorance, *most* of us—we creatures
of earth—are being bullied, abused, tortured, and killed by a
few of us who show no sign of voluntarily renouncing such
exploitation and colonization of naive, innocent, or defenseless
humans as well as other species, our planet, and the cosmos
we know.

These predators can't be stopped by physical force because
their unprincipled power is like steam, or spores, or a virus,
which can't be contained and will detect and follow any crack
in resistance and will seize every opportunity to establish
another colony to extend their empire. They can only be
controlled by the educated rejection of their false premises and
prurient appeals to the unscrupulous, the lazy, the naive, that
resides in each of us. They can be starved out of power by a
critical mass of people who understand that no one—not even
I—may exploit another without re-enforcing the foul order
we have today.

If I'm warm and comfortable I must do more than
recognize that fact and be grateful for these pleasures and
my good fortune. I must also make certain that those who
chop my firewood, plant and pick my food, build my house,
fabricate my clothing and furniture and shoes and jewelry and
rugs, mow my lawn and rake my leaves and shovel my snow,
clean my floors and walls and toilet, check out my groceries,
deliver my mail and my newspapers, tend my babies and teach

my children, process my waste, build and service my car and my computer, all have at least this basic level of well-being which I so enjoy and for which I am so grateful. If any of them doesn't share my clean, well-lighted condition due to exploitation by another person I must not profit by that fact.

I must speak up, speak out, challenge, denounce, and refuse to patronize or respect the CEO who takes the obscenely large salary while paying the sweeper or production line worker the minimum rate *tolerated* by law. I must not respect the faux do-good-ism of the economic colonialist/industrialist missionary who moves his factory around, in a corporate shell game, from one third-world country to another to exploit ever lower labor costs in order to pad his salary, his golden umbrella, or his bottom line while pretending to be participating in a world economy and to be responding to the mandates of his stockholders who wish him to hire trusting workers who end up selling their native skills and land and culture for a mess of promises quickly eaten—just because he can.

I must not respect those who have their way with the earth and other species, enslaving, clear-cutting, abusing, fouling, plundering, raping and pillaging, even if it is to provide me, or share-holders, or anyone else, with some imagined necessity. While I so piously appreciate all my blessings, I must keep in mind the fact that immorality by proxy is still immorality. The indirect, or trickle-down benefits of anyone's exploitive acts may not accrue to me.

Monday, January 8, 1996 — 10:50 p.m.

...by candlelight...

There are so many worlds in which it is possible to choose to live; some of them are delineated by light. A mercury vapor street light outside my window, in whose peach-colored aura fog droplets seem to swirl like fine snow driven by a fine movement of air, backlights a treetop. I miss snow; I love California but I'm homesick for Michigan.

…in the dark, by the light of my memory…

…the bowl of unbelievably satisfying cream of tomato soup after twenty-four hospital hours without food or water…the anesthesiologist hugging my upside-down head during a drug-induced pre-surgery crying jag…a nurses' aide delivering hot washcloths before lunch to my room-mate and me, when we were anchored to our beds with all four of our feet in stitches and casts…hearing "Karma Chameleon" in the operating room when my anesthesia got a little thin…. listening to Greg after his night shift as an emergency room medical technologist intern in an inner-city Detroit hospital, telling his choked story of trying to draw blood from the heel of a premature addicted baby delivered, during his shift, of its stoned mother…weeks after foot surgery recognizing the tailgating driver, who gave me the finger as he finally passed me on the freeway, as the orthopedic surgeon who had removed inches of bone from my feet…hormones rampaging madly through my sweating, bleeding, lactating, weeping body for insane days after the delivery of my baby girl and longing, pining, aching for the comfort of my own mother…post-partum depression…

Sunday, February 11, 1996

It's hard to believe that I'm writing outdoors, on the eleventh of February, clad only in tee-shirt and sweat pants. A pot of red tulips and another of blue crocuses share the slatted redwood table at my right. Coral-colored camellias sag from glossy green shrubs and lemons ripen quietly in a dwarf tree shading calla leaves rolling into the bright day. Slender daffodil leaves are eight inches tall in pots between a blooming white azalea and a jade plant bigger than a bushel. Boston ivy and spider plants sway in the gentle breeze as a senile rhododendron buds once again and shy ferns unfurl modestly in a corner. The place teems with fruit and flowers, green and growth, sunshine, birdsong, and sweet air.

Not entirely paradise, the top of the tall fence around this edenic place lists two feet farther southward than its base, courtesy of a fierce windstorm a month ago; repairs will be made when my landlady's name reaches the top of the long list of neighbors with similar damages.

Tuesday, February 20, 1996

A breezy, sunny day, a double-decaf-whole-milk-extra-hot-no-foam latte at hand, fading red tulips, finished blue crocuses, ripening lemons, leafing rose bushes, burgeoning alyssum, two callas unfurling, one modest daffodil (no partridges, no pear trees); what could be more hopeful and promising of blessings and summers to come? A bee is doing fly-bys, skimming the tulips and buzzing the daffodil. Sounding like a great airborne tractor, a plane moves heavily along a landing pattern—for San Jose airport a few miles south or for South San Francisco airport a few miles north?

I'm on telephone standby for jury duty this week so I'm not working. This is the first time I've ever been called so I hope I get a chance to serve.

Sunday, March 3, 1996

Thirsty from years in the tool shed
clay pots in a bucket of water
fizzle and sizzle and belch
alkali and cobwebs and salts.

Budding branches, like silver filigree with tiny jade chips at each twig end make it clear that spring is here.

I think it's safe now to conclude that natural light therapy has worked! I made it through the rainy season without having to consult a practitioner of any kind. I did have some problems with joint pains in my neck and shoulders, yet they never became severe enough to require more than take an occasional low potency homeopathic remedy and the usual two aspirin tablets daily. I'm still plagued with spurs and plates and miscellaneous bony outgrowths— called osteophytes, I just learned from an author who believes that natural light is nature's one and only remedy for disease, but I have finally discovered a promising therapy for them too.

Just as I've been thinking that perhaps the theories and therapies I've been using for the past four years have carried me as far as they will along my road to recovery; just as I've begun wondering if perhaps now I should begin incorporating other techniques that might be more creative, constructive and restorative rather than merely palliative or therapeutic, devices that might bring me to a greater than ever state of health, ease, comfort, energy, creative focus, I've run into a book that is a mother lode of explanations and plausible theories about why what I've done has worked so well, and about reasonable next steps.

The book is called *Food and Healing* and it's written by Annemarie Colbin, a certified health education specialist. It reads,

> Cattle grazing on the nightshade Solanum malacoxylon grow sick and deformed from an excess of vitamin D, which causes an increase of calcium and phosphate in the blood, a condition that leads to calcification of the aorta, kidneys, lungs, and the back of the neck. It may be relevant to note here that calcification of soft tissue—that is, the deposition of calcium (bone matter) in inappropriate places within the body—is possibly the most prevalent symptom in modern industrial cultures. Hans Selye has called it "the calciphylactic syndrome," and it is involved in arthritis, arteriosclerosis, coronary disease, cerebral sclerosis (senility), kidney stones, rheumatoid arthritis, chronic bronchitis, osteoporosis, lupus erythematosis, hypertension, and even certain forms of cancer.
>
> Nightshade foods may subtly remove calcium from the bones and deposit it in joints, kidneys, arteries, and other areas of the body where it does not belong. We can make sense out of this through the balance-of-opposites theory, in this case of the acid and the alkaline. In the meat-and-dairy diet, the acid-forming meat protein must be alkalized with minerals; the alkaloids in such nightshades as potatoes and tomatoes may be instrumental in keeping the alkalizing calcium dairy foods in solution, or pulling it out of blood or bones. If the process overshoots and too much calcium is liberated, the excess could indeed be redeposited in soft tissues as spurs, plaques, stones, or other calcifications. Vitamin D3 in the Solanum nightshades has been found to be involved in promoting calcification of body tissues.

Colbin says that eliminating all traces of nightshades has resulted in remissions of arthritic pain, RA, OA, bursitis, tennis elbow, gout, lower-back pain, muscle pain, and charley horse.

Wow, that's a lot! I remember hearing from an elementary school teacher that tomatoes and potatoes were originally regarded as poisonous by Europeans; I'm not surprised.

Colbin goes on,

> ...over thirty years ago, well before nightshades had fallen under any kind of suspicion, the macrobiotic regimen proposed by George Ohsawa recommended a total avoidance of these plant foods...coupled with the stricture against meat and milk products. Perhaps avoiding these foodstuffs, while increasing fresh vegetables, grains, and beans, might allow a disturbed calcium metabolism to calm down, and could lie behind the apparent success of macrobiotics in restoring joint flexibility and in shrinking spurs, plaques, and stones...

She also points out that natural light plays a vital role in the metabolism of calcium.

Obviously, full-spectrum light will be a daily consideration from now on—and meat and nightshades and dairy products will rarely (never say "never") darken my table again.

PART III

Honor Every Truth by Use

Proof, Sustained Recovery, and Passing It On

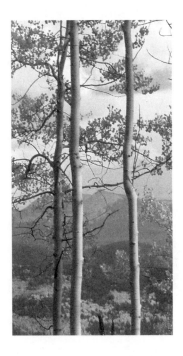

III

Honor Every Truth by Use

Sunday, September 1, 1996

THE CATS, MAJA AND LIDA, are languid and limp in the heat and move only to locate a cooler patch of earth, a lower-growing shrub. Markus N. Backus claws his way up the door screen and demands more than the walnut meat, more than the bit of pita bread I've already offered his squirrelly little self. He disdains a scrap of rice cake and disappears. He's looking better these days; for weeks he looked very scrawny and his once-magnificent tail looked so sorry and weedy I thought he might die, but he's back in all his gutsy, hairy glory.

Neko, a Siamese neighbor cat, slick and sable and sexy, slinks behind the camellias, the snail-ragged lilies, then vaults the fence to the world beyond. Her housemate, Finnegan, an orange-stripey, lose and lanky kind of Irish-looking cat, lopes behind, then plops under a geranium.

When the acanthus bloomed a month or more ago, it was pale and spindly but revived when I blessed it with buckets of fragrant compost from the backyard heap. Then squash leaves hung on their thick stems like limp parasols in the sun at the feet of the acanthus; their sturdy seeds resisted transformation into black earth in the compost and returned instead to life from the final remains of some winter dinner interred among the sodden leaves and grass clippings of a different season. The xeranthemum seeds, which I buried in a terra cotta pot filled with compost, sprouted then perished a week later in the scorching heat; now in their stead a valiant tomato plant pants in the heat, stumbles, and rises again to run another lap. Life following on life following on life.

WITH THIS ENTRY I will end and publish this account of my journey from long-term, progressive, debilitating rheumatoid arthritis to stable, limited, nuisance RA, via the long and circuitous route of standard medicine, which failed to halt or even slow the disease and condemned me to less than half a life, then several methods often collectively referred to as alternative medicine which have arrested but not cured the disease.

Because I used several alternative methods, sometimes simultaneously, sometimes overlapping, sometimes serially, I wouldn't know how to allocate credit but frankly, Scarlett, I don't give a damn.

What I *do* know is where I've been with this disease, rheumatoid arthritis. I've survived its depressions, limitations, exhaustion, pain, stiffness, and expense in terms of time and energy as well as dollars. I *do* know I've survived more than twenty years of the best standard treatment I and my insurance companies could buy but which did nothing to stop the disease and only made it worse.

And I *do* know where I am today; I'm functioning at about 90% of what was normal for me when I first developed this disease at age thirty-two in 1970. I still have the disease, and it does flare up when I do things that I know my body doesn't tolerate—mostly when I eat things I shouldn't eat. I haven't cured the disease; I have merely arrested it and eliminated the need to take dangerous, ineffective, expensive drugs and to have surgery every few years to try to do what the drugs couldn't accomplish. I still have the surgical scars and the deformity in my hands and feet, but they don't hurt and they're not getting worse. Even the spurs and plaques are finally disappearing now that I've finally discovered what causes them.

I *do* know that, because of what I've learned, both my son, now twenty-six, who has RA, and my daughter, twenty-four today, who has ankylosing spondylitis, have been able to keep their diseases under control, through alternative medicine, and to live very athletic lives. Kev is a rock climber, spelunker, cyclist, camper, runner, weight-lifter and Rain is a runner, swimmer, frisbee golfer, sea kayaker hospice-volunteer. Neither has taken standard medication; neither has any deformity. Both still have their diseases but they are easily and comfortably under control. I wish I had known at the beginning of my disease what they knew at the beginning of theirs...but that's a pretty common sort of wish...

Over the course of the four years since I abandoned allopathic treatment, I've fasted three times. I've consulted two homeopathic physicians in person and many others through their writings. I've self-prescribed homeopathic remedies off and on during the entire time. I've gone through several courses, of two to ten sessions each, of acupuncture, with two different practitioners. I've used oils, simple herbs, and herbal compounds from time to time. I've occasionally taken various vitamins and minerals.

I've changed my diet dramatically. I rarely eat meat. I occasionally have milk in decaffeinated coffee but not otherwise. I rarely eat cheese. I almost never eat the fare served in fast food places. I rarely eat saturated fats and rarely fry anything. In my own cooking I use only extra virgin olive oil and expeller-pressed organic canola oil. I eat organic produce and grains as much as possible.

Over these last four years, as well as during the years before that, I've also used meditation, imaging, and other mental and spiritual techniques which resuscitated failing hope time and time again.

In addition to all of these, I finally got around to consistently using a therapy I had read about in the early seventies but just never followed through on—light therapy. Light therapy is, I believe, what enabled me to get through the entire winter of '95-96 *without* resorting, in painful desperation, to seeing a practitioner, and natural light therapy was my final step into comfortable near-enough health.

Although I did start the winter, as usual, with an acceleration of shoulder and neck pain and stiffness and limitation, I committed myself, at around Christmas time, to spending an hour daily outdoors in natural light without my reading glasses. Sometimes that was pretty hard to do on rainy short winter days. Nonetheless, I tried to spend most weekday lunch hours outside. On rainy Saturdays and Sundays, I would simply stand outside under the overhang and let natural light enter my eyes. On a few occasions, when the rain was torrential, I sat in the car in the library parking lot with the window open for an hour or so.

I'm convinced that simply being in natural light for minimal periods each day is the reason I had no serious setback this past winter and the final increment that stabilized my recovery at 90% of what was normal for me at age thirty-two. More than that, I'm convinced that being in natural light so much during the dry seasons here was a major factor in my having been so well during these past four years; it is also the explanation, I believe, for my annual summertime improvement during my Michigan years.

I also credit natural light with eliminating a chronic depression, the depth of which I didn't realize until after it ended. Now that I think back, I realize that I was always better, physically and emotionally, during my Michigan summers, and my RA and depression would always worsen in winter.

Since I used them so unscientifically, I can't tell which, or what combination, of the therapies did what, that resulted in my sustained near-recovery. I wish now I *had* kept careful records, and used therapies one at a time, so I could now share *accurate* information with anyone who might want it. But perhaps that's just as well.

In using and combining medical therapies, including so-called standard therapies, I believe, even more strongly now, that the person seeking relief and cure must educate *herself,* thoroughly, before committing to *any* therapy, standard or alternative. I think it's imperative to stay aware not only of current scientific findings, but also of anecdotal information and, most important, of personal reactions and observations, evaluations, hunches, and speculations. I think it's especially important to avoid being carved up into little pieces to be treated separately. The 'doctor' should be healer, teacher, spiritual helper—one person—who treats not *parts* but *persons.*

From what I've learned from books and speakers and what I've observed myself, I've developed my own eclectic therapy and philosophy, but I'm finally beyond the stage where I accept any one person's—even my *own*—conclusions as gospel, that is, complete, universal, unchanging. I've finally learned that learning never stops, that I can learn something from everyone and everything from no one, and that I can pass on only the truths I've experienced.

My struggle with RA has not happened in a vacuum. It happened alongside and intertwined with family and philosophical and religious and spiritual crises as well as occupational struggles and discontent. In true chicken-or-egg fashion, I don't know which came first but I've always known that all my problems and challenges were inter-related. I've always known that there are no lines of demarcation among my physical, mental, spiritual, emotional, philosophical, behavioral, and social aspects. I've always known that the trick is to get everything flowing together in the same direction through *some* organizing principle, *some* philosophy, *some* paradigm, *some* acceptable myth; I've always known that the thought is mother to the fact. And I've known for a long time that *fear* is my downfall in health, work, faith. What I lacked more than anything was the courage, the moral resolve, to not *allow* my fears to govern my life.

I had no trust in my own assessments or the reasonableness of my desires to try other things. I often felt that I was an amateur acrobat flying without a net, a sailor of stormy seas with no life jacket. Looking back, I see that not only did I have no life jacket, I had no boat! I was trapped underwater and have only *now* broken the surface.

The main reason for that sense is the fact that I had no strong spiritual faith because I had no faith in the religious tradition in which I was raised nor in any I have since explored. I lacked the courage to invent my own spiritual system, to step off the well-trodden path of standard medicine, to defy the employment gods and try to do what I have wanted to do for as long as I can remember—or at least since I won a first-prize copy of *Alice In Wonderland* and *Through the*

Looking-glass in a Detroit News' "Young Writers Club" story contest when I was in grade three—to write for publication.

In 1992, I *chose* to be courageous. In 1992, I *made* myself courageous. I defied the authorities. I tried another way of treating my disease and succeeded. At the same time, I realized that faith, just like courage, is achieved by *fiat,* by *will.*

What it adds up to is this: I know I'm going to die sometime in the next seventy years or so and I don't know what comes next; but I do believe something does—this is all just too elaborate to be over so quickly. I don't know for sure whether there's a god who created the cosmos or what her rules for living are; but I do have a hunch and a hope and a wish and a belief that someone very grand hovers very close all the time and whispers guidance into my unconscious. In the absence of that certain knowledge but in the context of that faith, I must choose whether and how and why to live. As with most decisions in anyone's life, the decision must be made in the absence of inadequate information.

I do choose to live, for the moment at least, and I *choose* to *assume* that there is a god who is at *least* as good and kind, as loving, benevolent, helpful, creative, pleasant, and fun as I am in my best moments, those moments in which I feel I've added somewhat to my own fulfillment and joy and the fulfillment and joy of the cosmos. Therefore the style of living I want to choose is the one that seems to promise the most of those best moments.

I heard some best moment stories last night, at an orientation meeting of prospective California Court Appointed Special Advocates, from several advocates who have been in the program for some years. I learned that CASAs are trained volunteers who are appointed by judges to assure abused and neglected children don't fall through the cracks in an overburdened child protection system, that their needs are met during the time they are moving through the court system from temporary placement into safe and permanent homes. I learned that in 1995 there were 2,515 volunteers in California who served 4,150 children who may never have had even *one* adult who was truly committed to them individually.

This program asks for a commitment of ten to twenty hours per month to the child, in addition to all court hearings involving the child, as well as twelve advanced training hours per year. I can't decide whether I consider that a big commitment or not but I can't think of any program, outside of a good academic and moral education, that might help more to prevent the burgeoning social pathologies that threaten the world these days so I've signed up for the training program. That was a *very* good moment.

At last, my health is nearly normal and I can think more kindly about all the mainstream physicians whose efforts failed to sustainably help me and who, I finally realize, are neither the narrow-minded money-grubbing rogues I've often thought them nor the sainted heroes my mother believed them to be. At last and perhaps only for the moment, I'm content in my agnosticism and the faith I've crafted and, at last, I've slipped the surly bonds of unfulfilling work and am writing for a living.

"Evolutionary behavior is addictive and communicable," Jonas Salk says. "Conscious, self-propelled evolution is epidemic in society and its changes are spreading much more quickly than unconscious change."

"Honor every truth by use," says Ralph Waldo Emerson.

Suggested Readings

MOST OF THESE BOOKS were referred to specifically in the preceding pages; I've read them all along the way and each has contributed in some way to my physical, mental, or spiritual health. Believing as I do that each person will find a *unique* combination of teachers, I imagine that some of these might help inform you as well.

Burns, David. *Feeling Good: The New Mood Therapy.*
New York: Morrow 1980.
   Very helpful to a depressed person; contains explanations and exercises and offers much hope and encouragement. I wish I'd stumbled upon it when I was most depressed and didn't even know it—I might have recognized myself in its pages and saved myself some suffering.

Chaitow, Leon. *The Acupuncture Treatment of Pain.*
Rochester, VT: Healing Arts Press 1990.
   Mostly for the health professional, this book illustrates safe and effective methods for using acupuncture in pain relief. Includes a section on treatment of addiction.

Colbin, Annemarie. *Food and Healing.*
New York: Random House, Inc. 1996.
> Annemarie Colbin argues passionately that we must take
> responsibility for our own health and rely less on modern
> medicine; she shows that eating well is the first step toward
> better health. Draws upon an array of thinking, from ancient
> eastern to contemporary western, and shatters many myths
> about the standard American diet and food fads.

Cousins, Norman. *Anatomy of an Illness As Perceived by the Patient:
Reflections on Healing and Regeneration.*
New York: Norton 1979.
> Cousins took responsibility for his incurable illness and cured
> it in a very surprising way. A fascinating story, and well-told.

Cummings, Stephen and Ullman, Dana.
Everybody's Guide to Homeopathic Medicines.
Los Angeles: Jeremy P. Tarcher, Inc. 1991.
> The title says it all. A good first book.

Dossey, Larry.
Healing Words: The Power of Prayer and the Practice of Medicine.
New York: HarperCollins 1993.
> An eloquent and interesting book on healing power of
> faith, prayer, and spiritual practice. Reminds me of the old-
> fashioned saying, "More things are wrought by prayer than
> this world dreams of."

Emerson, Ralph Waldo.
Essays—First and Second Series, with introduction by Irwin Edman.
New York: Thomas Y. Crowell Co., Inc. 1951.
> To my mind, Emerson covers everything important in life
> and does so exquisitely.

Erasmus, Udo. *Fats That Heal, Fats That Kill.*
Burnaby, Canada: Alive Books 1993.
  "The complete guide to fats, oils, cholesterol and human
  health" reads the cover of this book that is filled with general
  information on the human body and its functions. Contains
  information, which I have not yet used, on the use of flax oil
  in the treatment of RA.

Ferguson, Marilyn. *The Aquarian Conspiracy.*
Los Angeles: J. P. Tarcher, Inc. 1980.
  Subtitled *Personal and Social Transformation in the 1980s,* this
  book is by no means stale or dated. Still a mind-blowing
  primer for the newly raised consciousness and full of hope
  and encouragement for the discouraged.

Geldard, Richard. *The Esoteric Emerson.*
Hudson, NY: Lindisfarne Press 1993.
  Commentary on the writings and ideas of my longest-term
  teacher, Ralph Waldo Emerson, who would be my guru if
  I—or he—believed in gurus. Geldard unfolds in detail the
  path of hearing and obeying intuitive whisperings which
  lead to authenticity and truth, and demonstrates that
  Emerson's path of the mind is also a path of the heart.

Grossman, Richard. *The Other Medicines.*
Garden City, NY: Doubleday & Company, Inc. 1985.
  Including history and practical applications of
  complementary medicines, and detailed illustrations, the
  author has assembled an easy-to-follow practical handbook
  for the preparation and application of many cultural
  medicines, including inhalants, teas, massages, exercises,
  breathing, stretching, etc. Includes an extensive bibliography
  with excellent annotations to help in deciding what to read
  next.

Harrison, John. *Love Your Disease.*
Santa Monica CA, Hay House, Inc. 1984.
> Harrison, an M.D. who has studied acupuncture, homeopathy, and naturopathy and, in his clinical practice, uses psychological techniques to treat physical complaints, asserts that disease is both self-created and self-cured.

Liberman, Jacob. *Light: Medicine of the Future.*
Santa Fe, NM: Bear & Company Publishing, 1991.
> How, when, and why light affects living things, especially humans. Very clear and easy to understand. Explains why sunlight is necessary to our well-being and why most fluorescent lighting, sunglasses, tanning lotions, and indoor lifestyles are harmful to it. Shows how not only our eyes, but our entire bodies, respond to light.

Lust, John. *The Herb Book.*
New York: Bantam Books, Inc. 1974.
> Contains clear illustrations and concise descriptions of the properties and uses of hundreds of medicinal and culinary herbs. A good basic book. I didn't use herbs enough to say how useful the format is.

Mander, Jerry. *In the Absence of the Sacred.*
San Francisco: Sierra Club Books 1991.
> An important book in my search for spiritual, as differentiated from physical, health. Discusses the failure of technology and the survival of the Indian Nations by the author of an earlier book arguing for the elimination of television!

McLaughlin, Corinne, and Davidson, Gordon.
Spiritual Politics: Changing the World from the Inside Out.
New York: Ballantine Books 1991.
From a metaphysical perspective, discusses such diverse
topics as the national health crisis and the Clarence Thomas
hearings. Asks the reader to re-examine her assumptions
about underlying principles and dynamics of our collective
political life. Insists that there is something important that
each of us can do here and now and at every moment.

Medicine Eagle, Brooke. *Buffalo Woman Comes Singing.*
New York: Ballantine Books 1991.
A spiritual autobiography of a Rainbow Warrior. Contains
several pages on fasting for spiritual reasons and gorgeous
illustrations by Prudence See as well as many enlightening
exercises and a wonderful myth about White Buffalo
Woman.

Moore, Thomas. *Care of the Soul.*
New York: HarperCollins, 1992.
Moore, a Jungian psychologist writes convincingly of the
sacredness of everyday life, of God present within the world
and the individual.

Ott, John. *Health and Light.*
Old Greenwich, CT: The Devin-Adair Co., 1973.
A fascinating story about the effects of natural and artificial
light on man and other living things by a professional time-
lapse photographer with RA who discovered by accident
how natural light improved his health.

Pelletier, Kenneth.
Mind As Healer, Mind As Slayer: A Holistic Approach to Preventing Stress Disorder.
New York: Dell Publishing Co. 1977.
Describes statistical personality-type-to-disease relationships, eerily accurate in my case. Describes the mechanics of disease in clear terms.

Pizer, Hank. *Guide to the New Medicine: What Works, What Doesn't.*
New York: William Morrow and Company, Inc. 1982.
Examines the growing popularity of alternative healing methods among those who believe that ours is an overmedicated prescription culture and that the medications used to combat illness often pose more of a threat than the illness itself. A balanced presentation of a wealth of information, favorable and unfavorable, on alternative medicine. Evaluates specific alternative healing practices and practitioners; reveals the good they have done as well as the charlatanism that lurks in these—and every—type of medical practice. Explores whether non-allopathic healers rely on faith alone or whether their treatments have scientific value.

Robbins, John. *Diet For a New America.*
Walpole, NH: Stillpoint Publishing 1987.
How food choices affect health, happiness, and the future of life on earth. Decries our dependence upon other animals as food, and the inhumane and unhealthy conditions under which meat animals are raised.

Rogers, Eric N. *Fasting: The Phenomenon of Self-Denial.*
Nashville, TN: Thomas Nelson, Inc., Publishers 1976.
A dispassionate account of fasting as a means to good health, as manifestation of the sporting instinct, for scientific

research, as attention-getting device; for religious cleansing, commemoration, penance, and preparation for the appearance of a spiritual guide. 160 fascinating pages.

Shelton, Herbert. *Fasting Can Save Your Life.*
Tampa, FL: American Natural Hygenic Society, Inc. 1991.
The best place to start. The most complete and convincing book I found on the subject of fasting. I didn't follow all of Shelton's admonitions but I did know what they were.

Simonton, O. Carl and Simonton, Stephanie Matthews, and Creighton, James.
Getting Well Again: A Step-By-Step Self-Help Guide to Overcoming Cancer for Patients and Their Families.
Los Angeles: J. P. Tarcher, Inc. 1978.
Written primarily for cancer patients but includes useful imaging exercises and an excellent exercise on forgiveness.

Tierra, Michael. *Planetary Herbology.*
Twin Lakes, WI: Lotus Press 1992.
Readable reference guide to hundreds of medicinal herbs available in the west, cross-referenced to Chinese and Ayurvedic systems of herbal therapy. Beautifully hand-illustrated.

Ullman, Dana. *Discovering Homeopathy.*
Berkeley: North Atlantic, 1988.
An well-organized and interesting introduction to the science and art of homeopathic medicine. More than an summary, this is a good second book after *Everybody's Guide to Homeopathic Medicines.*

Van Over, Raymond. *Total Meditation.*
New York: Collier Books, 1978.
> A careful explanation of what meditation is, how it works, and what it offers. Includes a great section on how meditation actually affects the brain and the body. Includes specific instructions on Zen, Yoga, T'ai Chi, TM, and other forms of meditation.

Vithoulkas, George. *The Science of Homeopathy.*
New York: Grove Weidenfeld 1980.
> A scholarly and in-depth, yet readable, near-textbook outlining both the theory and practice of homeopathy.

Weil, Andrew. *Natural Health, Natural Medicine.*
Boston: Houghton Mifflin Company 1990.
> A comprehensive manual for wellness and self-care, stressing prevention of illness. Has a concise section on fasting and other simple measures. Includes good sections on vitamins and supplements, herbals, and home remedies for common ailments. Clear and easy to read, yet detailed and complete. Specifies precise steps to take toward better health.

Whitaker, Julian. *Dr. Whitaker's Guide to Natural Healing.*
Rocklin, CA: Prima Publishing 1995.
> Contains natural remedies, alternative therapies, and preventive techniques for specific conditions.

Index

From:

NAME _____

ADDRESS _____

CITY, STATE, ZIP _____

NUMBER OF BOOKS

Please send _____ copies of
Finding Ways at $19.95 each.

Total: $_____

SALES TAX

Please add 7.75% ($1.55) for each copy
mailed to a California address.

Total sales tax: $_____

SHIPPING

Please add $3.55 for the first copy
and $1.25 for each additional copy

Total shipping: $_____

TOTAL CHECK OR MONEY ORDER ENCLOSED: $_____

(Sorry, no credit cards accepted)

Please Mail Order To:

Synchrony Publishing

PO Box 60205 ❧ Palo Alto, California 94306